PURIFY

REJUVENATE

RITUAL

CLARITY

CALM

Bathe

Suzanne Duckett

with Georgina Rodgers

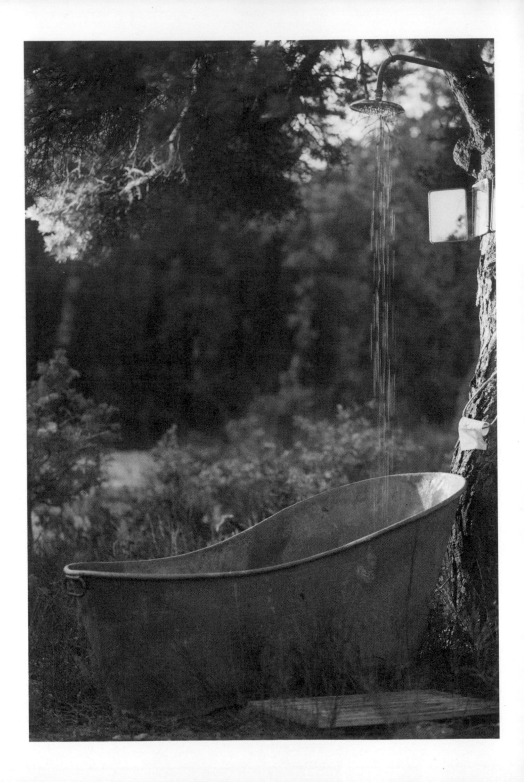

PURIFY

REJUVENATE

RITUAL

CLARITY

CALM

Bathe

Rediscover the Ancient Art of Relaxation

Suzanne Duckett

with Georgina Rodgers

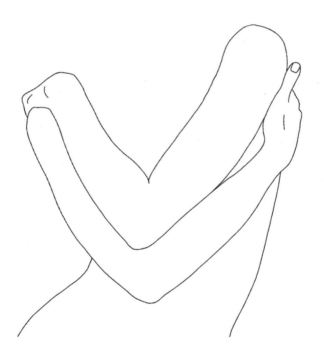

To my mum

I loved every one of those warm baths you ran for me as a nipper and can still feel the sense of security and love when you wrapped me up in a warm, soft, fluffy towel afterwards (I upgraded Mr Matey though!).

To my husband Andy

Thanks for keeping us in stock of 25kg sacks of Epsom salts. For that reason alone you are my rock star!

To my daughter Tallulah

Thank you baby girl for your interest in my work and mutual love of bathing, spas and wellness adventures that we have experienced together at home and around the world. Long may they continue.

To my dogs Rosco & Ruben

I know you think you hate baths, but you love them really and you are much better housemates after a quick dip. Trust us.

CONTENTS

INTRODUCTION

10

Our long love affair with bathing 16

The watery world of the womb 21

The joy of solo time 23

A brief history of bathing:
Where did it all begin? 24

The world's most amazing bathtubs 28

Bathtime Brainwaves 30

The politics of naked bathing,
at home and abroad 32

The christening effect: The ultimate blessing –
dunking in the name of God 37

Companionship and communal bathing:
It's in our DNA 40

British Bathing 45

Wild bathing: Hidden dips in rivers,
lakes and waterfalls 46

[ONE]
Purify

49

Power baths 54

Four detoxing bath recipes for
improved health 58

Five restorative recipes for body and mind 66

The simple beauty of Japanese onsen 74

Japanese etiquette: How to onsen 78

Sentos vs onsen 80

What is 'skinship'? 83

It's not just humans who love onsen! 85

How to bathe Japanese-style 86

Excerpt from Yasunari Kawabata's
Snow Country 88

A simple bathtime breathing exercise to purify
the mind and relax the nervous system 90

Five of the best natural spas for a soak 93

Bathtime Brainwaves 96

Some like it hot! Inside the sauna 99

Bare sauna facts: Finnish sauna etiquette 102

Take a cold plunge: Ice-bathing
after a sauna 103

Feeling lonely? Take a bath 104

[TWO]
Rejuvenate

107

Bathing: The Science 112

What is a Turkish hammam? 116

How to get the hammam glow at home 119

Is taking a hot bath as good as exercise? 122

Thalassotherapy for healing 124

Bathtime yoga: Five bathtime stretches 126

Bathing through the seasons 128

Baths with a difference: Weird baths from
around the world 136

Bathtime Brainwaves 140

Why do we go wrinkly in the bath? 143

[THREE]

Ritual

145

Reframe your bathtime: How to create your own personal bathing ritual 151

Seven easy ways to spruce up your bathroom 153

No pain, no gain: A guide to Russian Banyas 157

Are we short-changing our bathtime? 159

Jimjilbang: The South Korean one-stop shop to relaxation 160

Jimjilbangs: The how-to 162

Top ten bathing accessories and why they matter 164

Bathtime Brainwaves 166

Music to have on your bathtime playlist 168

Five ways to read in the bath (without getting your book wet!) 170

A guide to eating and drinking in the bath 172

[FOUR]

Clarity

175

The blue mind: Creativity and problem solving in the bath – why do we find clarity when bathing? 180

Five bathtime exercises to fuel creative thinking 185

'Diplomacy without a tie': The Finnish art of networking in the nude 186

Bathtime Brainwaves 188

Digital detoxing: Technology has no place in the bathroom! 191

A simple bathtime breathing exercise to feel energised and focused 192

Shinrin-Yoku: The art of bathing in the forest 194

Soul-cleansing: How to bathe well in the forest 196

Romantic poetry and an encounter with the sublime 198

'On Revisiting the Sea-Shore, After Long Absence' by Samuel Taylor Coleridge 200

[FIVE]

Calm

203

Three DIY recipes to soothe, calm and beautify the skin 208

A bath before bedtime: Why is a bath the perfect wind-down activity? 215

Aromatherapy: Natural healing through bathing 216

Six healing aromatherapy bath rules 222

Twenty healing natural ingredients and how they could help you 224

Weightless: Discover the hidden joys of flotation 229

Gong baths – What are they? 231

Take a moment: Relaxation after the bath 232

Bathtime Brainwaves 234

Raising the bar: The simple soap 236

Excerpt from 'The Prelude' by William Wordsworth 240

Final Thoughts 242
Index 246
Acknowledgements 252
Picture credits 254

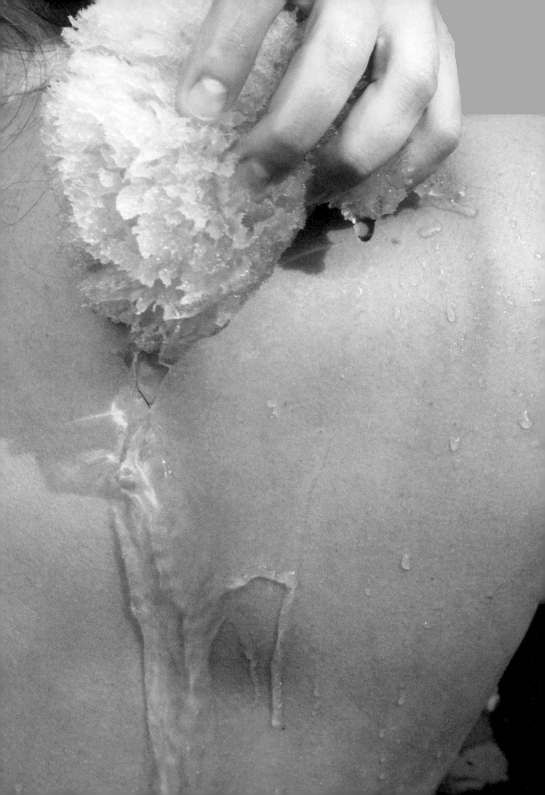

Bathe

/bath/ *verb*

to take a bath

to become immersed
or absorbed

INTRODUCTION

There is simply nothing like soaking in a steamy, aromatic bath to unwind both body and mind at the end of a long, hard day; it is a moment to recline, repose, lie back and close our eyes.

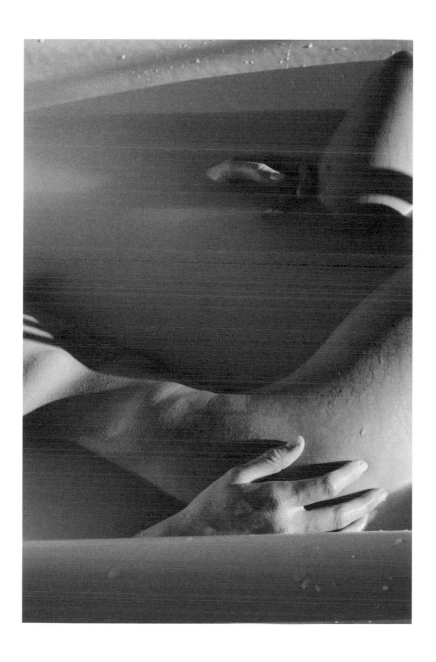

11 Bathe

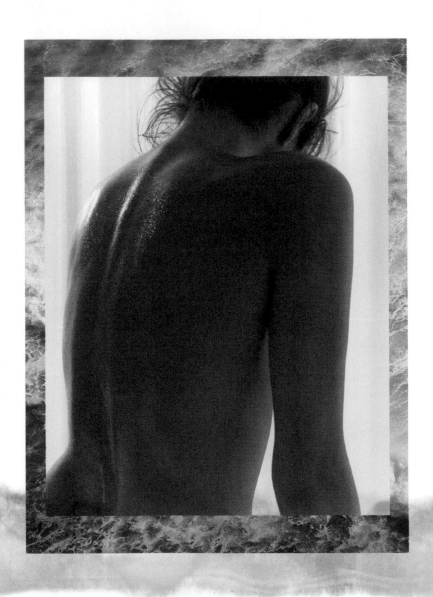

12 Bathe

There are few pleasures to rival this rare, innate idleness and exquisite stillness. While the wellness world whirs at a hundred miles an hour with the latest treatments and practices, the humble bath has stood the test of time. Baths are the ultimate equaliser and the most accessible and universal form of self-care for both men and women, with the remarkable power to instantly transform how we look and feel.

This simplicity makes taking a bath more needed than ever before, and since the beginning of time, baths have been used for their healing and revitalising properties. Cleopatra is said to have preserved her great beauty by bathing in the milk of 700 lactating donkeys each day, Winston Churchill insisted on having two hot baths a day to de-stress from the pressures of being a wartime leader and Freddie Mercury came up with the idea for 'Crazy Little Thing Called Love' while taking a dip! In the present day, everyone from A-list celebrities to politicians are tuning into the transformative power of the daily bath. Baths evoke varying emotions in different people. For some, they are a weekly exercise in self-indulgence and a luxurious personal ritual with twinkling candles, oils or salts poured into the water and a glass of wine to hand. For others, a daily wash while reading a crinkled book is part of their wind-down schedule before bed. For many, having a bath is the only time in the day when they can simply shut the door on the world and be on their own; it is an indulgent moment of privacy and solitude.

There are many types of baths and bathing rituals around the world and not all involving immersion in water. There's also steam generated from sizzling hot coals, dry heat and even immersion in nature (forest bathing) and sound. Humans have been shedding their clothes, along with their daily worries for thousands of years to seek escape and find a sense of rejuvenation and renewal. Public bathing is also about a sense of community, and without symbols that signify status or class, there is a sense of equality, kinship and oneness. Japanese society, for example, has the term 'skinship' for the bond created in villages and small social groups by sharing a bathhouse.

Bathing is having a timely resurgence, creating a new and much-needed movement. It is a shortcut to finding peace and calm as a way to de-stress and be mindful. Being immersed in water liberates the body, allowing an escape from the distractions of daily life, and it has been repeatedly shown that is it a great way to unwind. But it is much more than that. It has a host of fantastic, health-boosting scientific benefits that cannot be underestimated; it can stimulate the immune system, improve sleep, help skin conditions, boost circulation and heart health, benefit muscles and joints, and balance hormone levels.

Bathe is for readers everywhere, of every age; whoever you are and wherever you live, work and play, this book is for you. Designed to be read in the bath, as well as elsewhere of course, it features a host of practical take-away self-care tips to set you on a bathing journey to help heal both mind and body. Featuring the science, history and theories around bathing, it also includes inspirational quotes, poems, short meditations, creative exercises and practical tips so you can get the most from your baths. From how to create a sumptuous Japanese bathing experience at home, through to why people have their best creative brainwaves in the bath, this book is the ultimate compendium of bathing. Devour at leisure and slowly, just like the very essence of bathing itself.

Join the bathing movement at lovetobathe.com

'While the wellness world whirs at a hundred miles an hour with the latest treatments and practices, the humble bath has stood the test of time'

Our long love
affair with bathing

'Water is the driving force
of all nature'

Leonardo da Vinci

'Get in the bath!' How many times do you remember hearing those words as a child, or as a parent, how regularly do you instruct your little ones to hop into the bubbles? Often there is resistance to get in but once the bath works its magic, there is a resistance to get out! Even from childhood, we use bathtime to do more than clean our bodies, we use it to immerse in the here and now, allowing the wonder of water to wash away our troubles; we instinctively understand the healing and restorative powers of the bath.

Bathing is a central pillar of not only health and wellness but of families and many communities, who bathe together as a form of bonding and kinship. Bathing also takes on a symbolic and ritualistic quality. With its relationship to baptism and other cleansing rites, bathing has long been seen as a ceremonial, ritualistic and innate act of humankind.

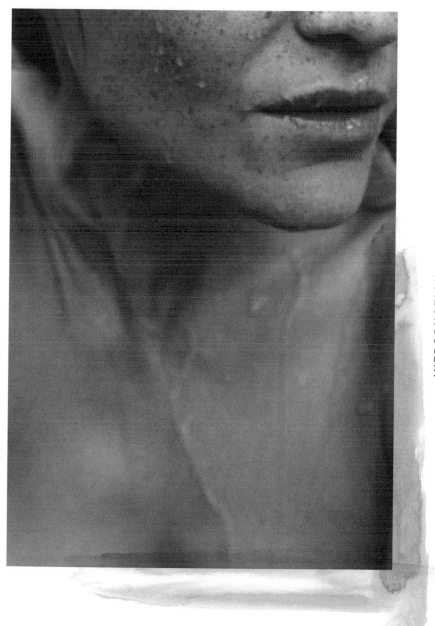

17   Bathe

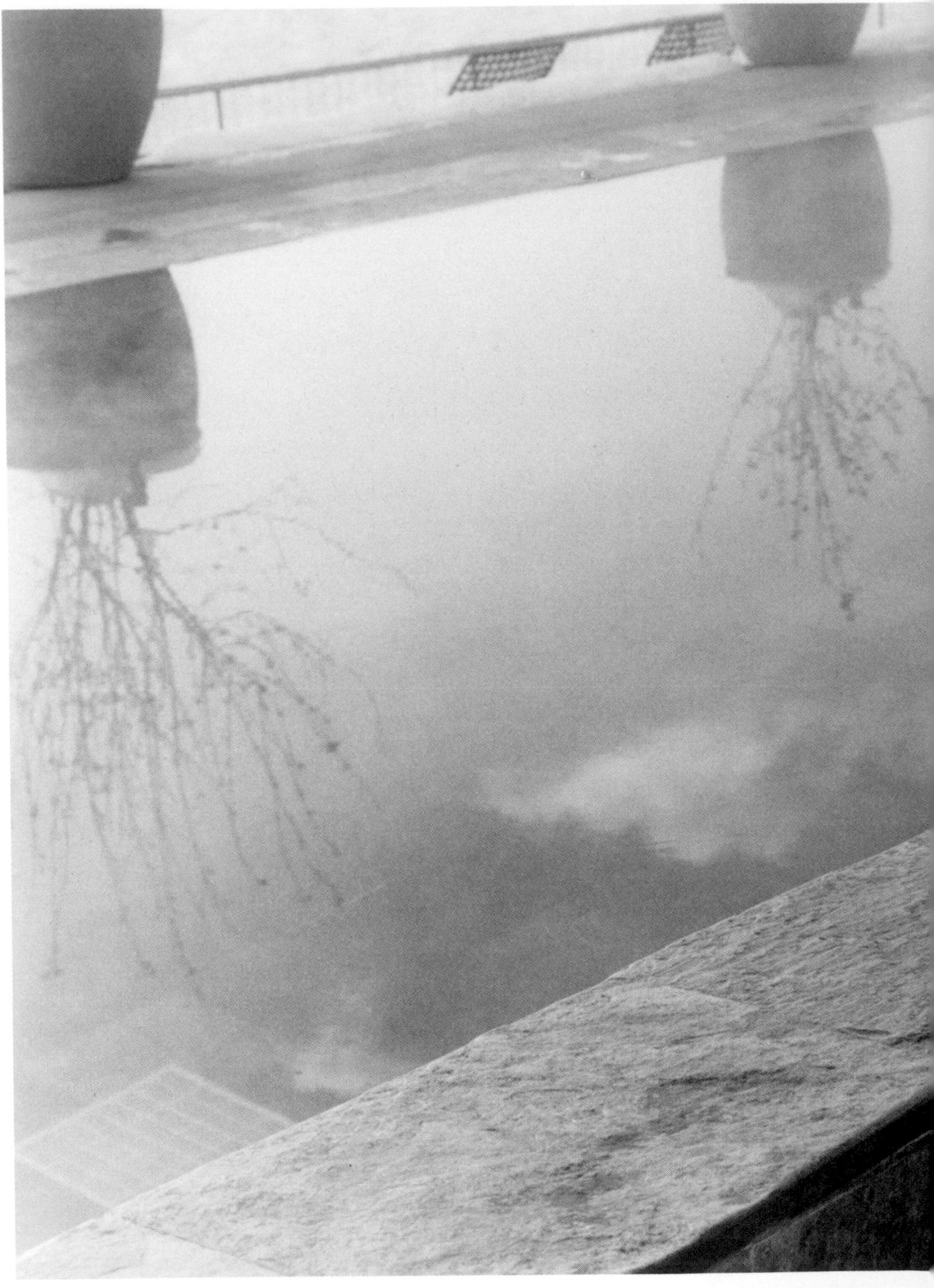

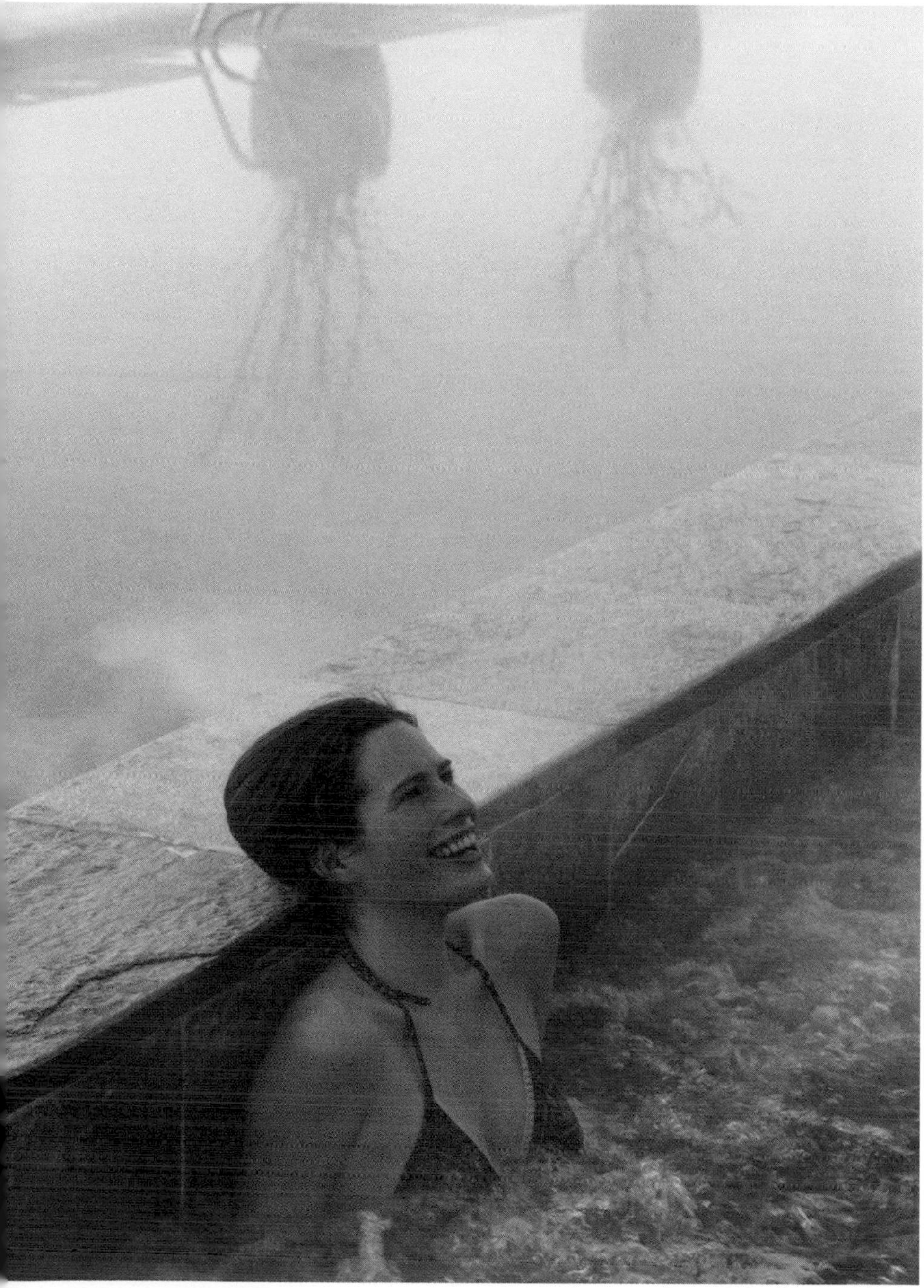

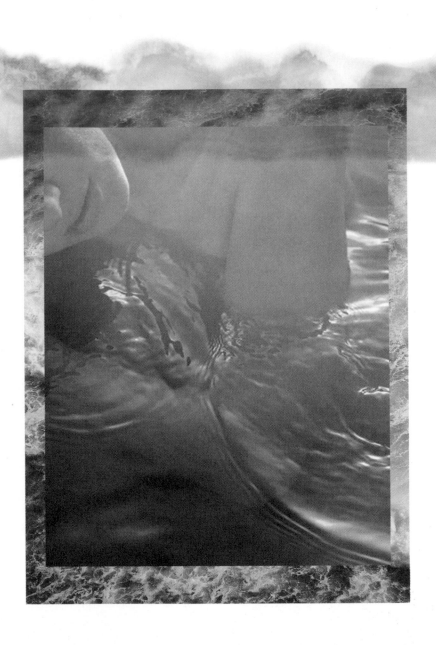

20   Bathe

The watery world
of the womb

We start our life and our bathing journey floating around in water; it is innate to us.

On a subconscious level, the floating sensation and soothing quality of a bath is said to remind us of the months we spent curled contentedly in our mothers' warm and watery wombs. Just like a growing baby *in utero*, baths offer us a wonderfully effortless combination of isolation, quiet and comfort, mimicking the sacrosanct security of the womb. There is simply no part of daily life more akin to being back there, and in a bath we find ourselves again contained in an enclosed place, wallowing in warm water away from the troubles and muffled sounds on the other side of the bathroom door. Naked, calm, mind clearing, body softening …

INTRODUCTION

The joy of solo time

Who has time to simply wallow and luxuriate in the bath?

The bath might be a central and essential part of any home but many favour a power shower over time in the tub. Fast, economical and practical, you can pop in and out of a shower in just a few minutes. They have the perfect functional purposefulness that is exactly compatible with the current speed and productivity-obsessed world in which we live.

Baths, however, take us back to a different mindset and age; slower, more contemplative and methodical, they are a positively analogue way of cleansing and relaxing. For busy people across human history, a bath might be the only time of peace, privacy and introspection in their week; it is a remedy to the bombardment of noise, chatter and rush of their life.

Hang up your 'Do Not Disturb' sign and embrace the solitude.

INTRODUCTION

A brief history of bathing: Where did it all begin?

It might be easy to imagine that before modern times people never bathed regularly, but throughout history many cultures have created their own bathing rituals for spiritual, religious, therapeutic or social reasons.

- **1,500 BC**: In Ancient Egypt, the people were very fond of bathing rituals and would cleanse themselves with a dip in a canal or river, or wash their hands, faces and feet in water basins. The Ancient Egyptians made their own cosmetics, including a soap made of paste or clay, which was often scented with oils. They believed that the cleaner and more well-oiled a person was, the closer they were to the Gods.

- **500–300 BC**: In Ancient Greece the men would participate in sports and public games in gymnasiums – or 'gymnos' – in the nude. Afterwards, servants would pour cold water out of jugs over them, setting the wheels in motion for the modern shower.

- **Roman Era**: The Ancient Romans first identified the medicinal benefits of regular baths, and communal bathhouses were the heart of Roman towns. People would socialise, exercise and relax in rooms of differing temperatures before bathing together. Later, when the Roman Empire collapsed in AD 1453, many bathhouses and private bathing facilities fell into disrepair.

- **AD 700:** Despite growing disapproval from the Church, many people still attended bathhouses to socialise and relax. There are numerous depictions from this time of people together, eating and drinking and being entertained by musicians while bathing. Bathhouses were also hedonistic places where sex and prostitution went on.

- **AD 710:** The origins of Japanese bathhouses can be traced back to Buddhist temples in India, and baths were found in temples, used initially only by priests for religious reasons. Sick people gradually gained access as well and bathed as a form of healing.

- **1340s–50s:** By this time, bathhouses had fallen out of fashion. People thought that illnesses could be spread via open pores and that dirt would block the disease from entering their bodies. They bathed privately in their homes according to their status and wealth. In 1351, King Edward III upgraded his bathroom to contain the ultimate luxury – hot and cold running water for his tub.

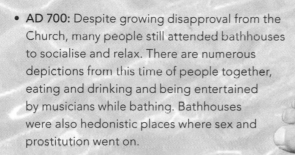

25   Bathe

- **1767**: The first shower as we would recognise it today was patented by London stove maker William Feetham. This invention pumped water into a basin above the bather's head, before they pulled a chain that would release the cold water. The same water would then be used over and over again!

- **1846:** An Act of Parliament granted local authorities the power to establish bathing facilities and offered them loans to do so. Many new baths, now recognised as swimming pools, opened and they were rich in detail and had opulent interiors.

- **1860s–90s:** The idea that the spread of disease could be prevented with good sanitation and bathing had taken hold and, in many homes, people started to bathe regularly. Some homes had bathrooms installed but many still relied on tin tubs for their weekly wash. It was common for the whole family to share one tub of water, with the most important person (the father) using it first, followed by the mother and children.

- **1900–50s:** Towards the end of the century, indoor plumbing and washing facilities became a legal requirement. Showers were also introduced during this period and bathrooms were beginning to be seen as a source of pride for the home, featuring en suites and there was a demand for colour and tiles.

'Throughout history
many cultures
have created their
own bathing
rituals for spiritual,
religious, therapeutic
or social reasons'

The world's most amazing bathtubs

Bathtubs have always been viewed by many as sumptuous works of art.

The first tub ever recorded in 1,700 BC in the Queen's apartments at the Palace of Knossos in Crete exuded indulgence, luxury and elegance. The 'tub'-like vessel measured just five foot and was terracotta in colour and decorated with watery reeds. It was filled and emptied by hand but the palace also contained the height of modern comfort: flushing lavatories, sinks and fresh water, which was carried from an aqueduct, via terracotta pipes.

If you love sinking right down to your chin, a soaking tub made of wood or stainless steel might be your dream bath. But nothing spells luxury quite like a sunken bathtub, a free-standing number or even a tub made from exquisite marble or nickel and brass.

Combine an elegant bathtub with an epic view and you can take bathing to another level. From glass-bottomed bathtubs in the Maldives and outdoor hot tubs with dreamy, colourful views of the Northern Lights in Iceland, through to outdoor safari tubs in the African bush, where you can watch elephants slosh around a waterhole or other wild animals roam free and infinity baths stretching into the clear azure ocean in the Caribbean, perhaps it's time to start thinking about the bath and its view next time you book a holiday?

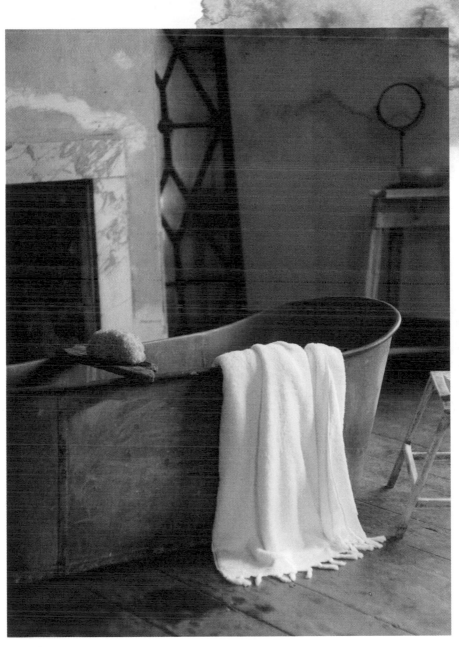

29   Bathe

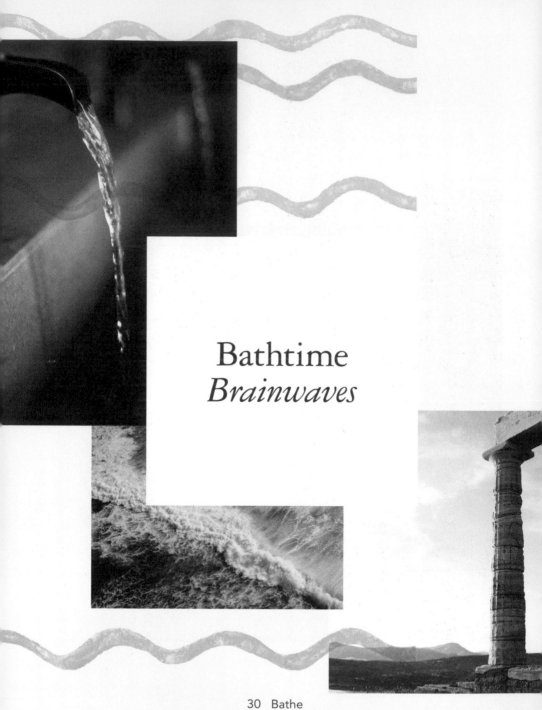

Bathtime
Brainwaves

Many of the greatest minds in history have had their best brainwaves while having a soak.

[ARCHIMEDES]
287–212 BC

The Greek mathematician and scientist made one of the most famous discoveries in history – the 'Eureka!' moment – by calculating the volume of an irregular shaped object when he noticed the water rose when it was placed in the bathtub. This is known as Archimedes' principle.

[BENJAMIN FRANKLIN]
1706–90

One of the Founding Fathers believed that nudity was good for you and he took regular 'cold' air baths for his health, a practice that was considered a tonic at the time. He would open the windows of his home and sit in front of a window, allow the air to circulate around him and work for up to an hour.

The politics of naked bathing, at home and abroad

We all pop into the world naked but as we grow up, our ideas and customs around nudity change due to the culture and time we live in, our parents and our religion. When, where and how many clothes we wear seems to matter more than you might think, depending on where you live.

In countries where public bathing is rare, such as in the UK, Australia and the US, it is strictly swimsuit territory and the vast majority of people wash privately alone at home. Bathing tends to fast forward to showering much earlier in life, saving baths for special occasions or for when we feel like having a long soak. Generally, people are not that comfortable being naked around each other and getting clean is more of a functional act in the shower.

For some communities, wearing nothing but a smile is quite normal. Germany, Austria and many Eastern countries have long held a relaxed attitude towards nakedness, and though in recent years there has been a decline in nudity in the open air, public baths and saunas are considered clothes-free environments (mainly for hygiene reasons because swimwear is thought to harbour bacteria). Modesty is left outside and most public baths are mixed and even where men and women enter through separate changing rooms, everyone comes together when immersing themselves, while having great conversation in the baths. Being naked in front of strangers is the stuff of nightmares if you are not used to it but in here any swimsuit-clad bathers become the oddity.

The Japanese, Turks and Scandinavians also enjoy communal bathing as a means of socialising. In Japan, where women enjoy the longest life expectancy in the world, communal activities, including bathing, are said to play an important role in maintaining the health and happiness of the ageing population. This is in marked contrast with the UK, where we tend to hide nudity, particularly as we age.

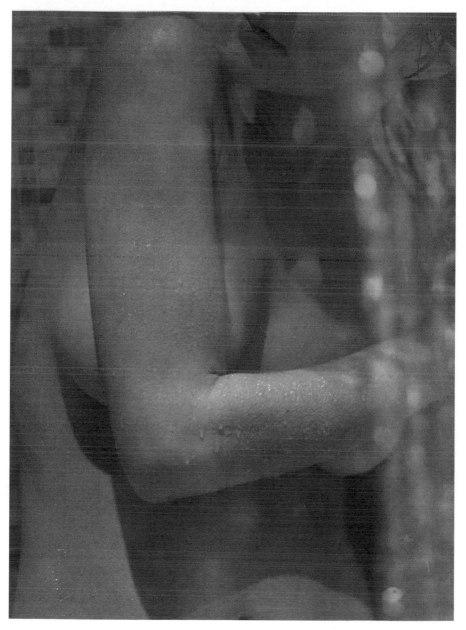

33 Bathe

Do you bathe with other family members? In the West, this is very much an individual thing and, after childhood, generally unusual. In the privacy of Japanese family homes, bathing naked together for a long time is commonplace. Many homes have high-tech bathtubs with control panels to keep the water warm and at a consistent temperature, as well as a multitude of other functions. We all need to bathe, so the Japanese do not make it a solitary activity, and like the public bathhouses, they use the home bath for relaxing, not cleansing. Some Japanese children continue bathing with their parents until high school and beyond.

Perhaps more surprising for those living in Western cultures is the fact that adolescents take baths with parents of the opposite gender – fathers bathing with daughters and mothers soaking with sons. Bathing together is associated with confidences and emotional closeness and one undisclosed boys' private school survey even suggested that those children who bathed with their mothers tended to achieve better grades.

'In Japan, communal activities, including bathing, are said to play an important role in maintaining the health and happiness of the ageing population'

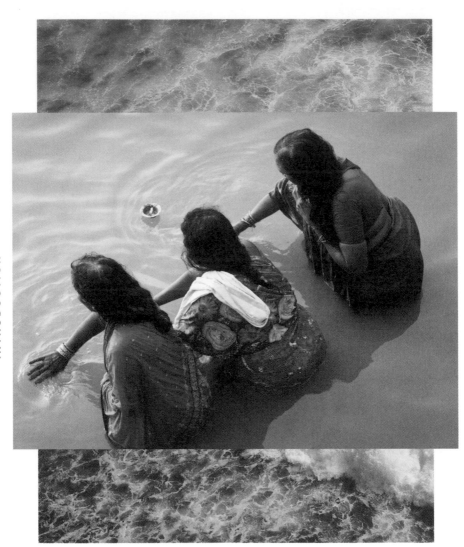

36   Bathe

The christening effect:
The ultimate blessing – dunking
in the name of God

Water is one of the most common elements in nature and is a central building block of life.

Alongside the air we breathe, water and the act of bathing plays a central role in many religions because of the belief that it has the ability to purify and cleanse, both spiritually and externally. Religions pay homage to the fact that water has the power to create and destroy and without it, there is no life.

- **Buddhism:** The offering of water within Buddhist shrines symbolises the desire to nurture calmness, clarity and purity of mind and body. Water is also said to epitomise the 'sweet nectar' of Buddha's teachings, nourishing spirituality.

- **Christianity:** The use of water and what it symbolises runs through all Christian churches and sects. It is a sign of purity and represents cleansing from sin. Every baptism in the Bible was by immersion under water, including the baptism of Jesus by John the Baptist. Holy water, used during baptisms, signifies that life is given to man by God and identifies us with Christ's death, burial and resurrection.

- **Hinduism:** Water is believed to have spiritually cleansing powers and to all Hindus, water is sacred, especially rivers. There are seven sacred rivers and they are thought to be a great equaliser, where distinctions of caste do not mean anything as people bathe and immerse themselves because all their sins fall away. Water is an essential feature in nearly all Hindu ceremonies.

- **Islam:** In the Koran, water is credited with the sacred qualities of life-giving, purifying and sustaining. The words 'we made from water every living thing' emphasise its central role. Muslims must be pure before prayer and some mosques have a courtyard with a clear pool of water, while others have them situated outside the walls for completing ablutions.

- **Judaism:** Ritual bathing in Judaism is seen as a way of maintaining purity. The bath used for the purpose of ritual conversion is called the mikveh and it is designed to ritually cleanse a person from deeds of the past. In the days of the ancient Temple in Jerusalem, the mikveh was used by all Jews who wanted to enter the precincts of the Sanctuary. Unmarried women would immerse themselves in the mikveh prior to their wedding and again following their menstrual periods or after childbirth. This ritual has decreased in modern times but many Jewish women still practise this.

- **Sikhism:** Like Hinduism, water plays a key role in prayer and is thought to purify the mind and body. A sarovar is the large pool of water, located near gurdwaras (Sikh temples). Originally they were built for practical purposes such as fresh water supply, but now they are used primarily by pilgrims for washing feet or performing sacred ablutions. Some sarovars are believed to have curative properties because of the continual prayers recited nearby.

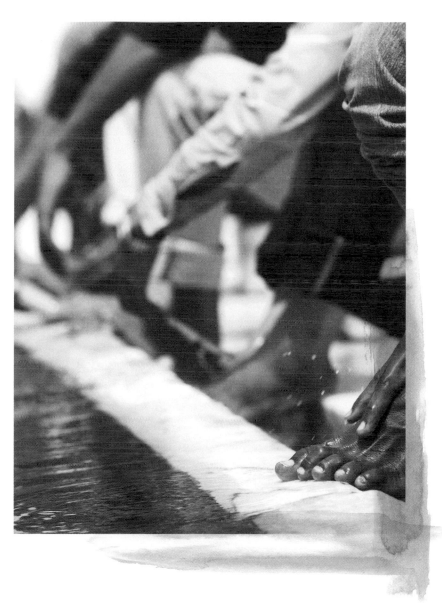

39 Bathe

Companionship and communal bathing: It's in our DNA

Public bathing, which is thought to be as old as humanity itself, is not just about health and cleansing; it is about pleasure, socialisation and a feeling of community.

Dating back as early as the Neolithic period, where nomadic tribes would soak in natural hot springs that they stumbled upon and relieve themselves from the cold, bathhouse culture is integral in many societies and has adapted as social norms and traditions change.

THE GREAT BATH

The oldest bathhouse in the ancient world was built with baked brick around 2,500 BC and is located in the lost city of Mohenjo-daro. Excavated in the early 1900s by archaeologists in present-day Pakistan, many believed it was used as a temple because bathing and religion are so closely connected at the site.

ROMAN THERMAE

Bathing was a very commonplace activity in Roman culture for both rich and poor and was a place for fun, friendship, courtship, business meetings and more. Built on lavish hot springs, in many ways these baths resembled modern-day spas, with changing rooms, gyms, rooms of differing temperatures, meditation rooms and exercise areas. Sometimes they were segregated by gender, but many were mixed. They were lavishly decorated and some could accommodate up to 6,000 people at one time. Many brought servants with them to give them massages and serve food. Healers would also reside in these bathhouses and treat people with gems, herbs and oils.

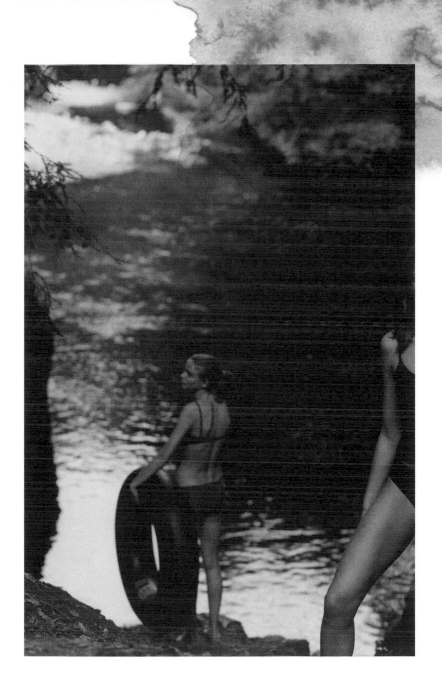

41 Bathe

TURKISH HAMMAM

As well as the Romans and Greeks, the Turks created a hot bathing experience that is still known as a Turkish steam bath or 'hammam'. The most impressive examples of these no-expense-spared, lavish and artistically-decorated houses are found in Istanbul, the capital of the Ottoman Empire and former capital of the Byzantine Empire. In the beginning only men were welcomed in hammams, but eventually women could bathe here too. Open from sunrise to sunset, major life events were celebrated here and bathing rituals featured as part of births and weddings.

RUSSIAN BANYA

Steam baths have long been part of ancient Slavic culture and steam baths in wooden bathhouses were popular throughout Eastern Europe. Banyas have been an important part of Russian people's lives because, according to folklore, they provided miraculous healing. The word 'banya' derives from the Latin *balneum*, which means 'to chase out pain' and in banyas, people are warmed at intense heats before lashing themselves with tree branches to boost circulation and then hopping into cold rivers and ponds. Banyas were associated with a healthy way of life and prices were kept low, so they could welcome as many people as possible.

JAPANESE ONSEN

The Japanese tradition of bathing in outdoor natural hot springs dates back to when Buddhism spread throughout the country. Dogo Onsen, located in Matsuyama, is said to have a 3,000-year history. The discovery of some remote and beautiful onsen was attributed to ancient hunters, who stumbled across them while pursuing their prey. Buddhist monks were key in popularising the onsen, and on their arrival in Japan in 552 BC, they integrated the ritual of bathing into their daily lives. Soon, onsen became a place for all, welcoming aristocracy and peasants alike.

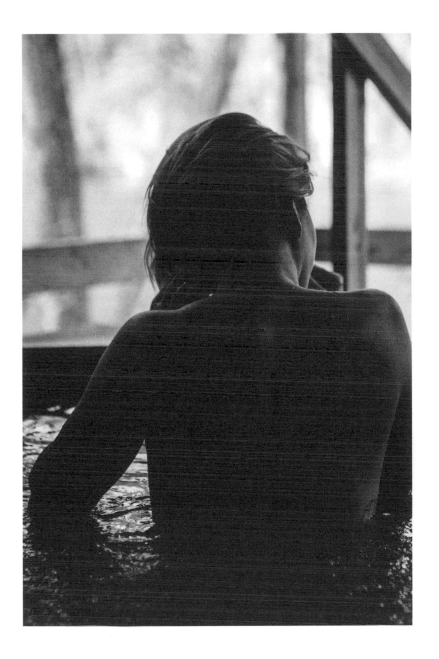

43   Bathe

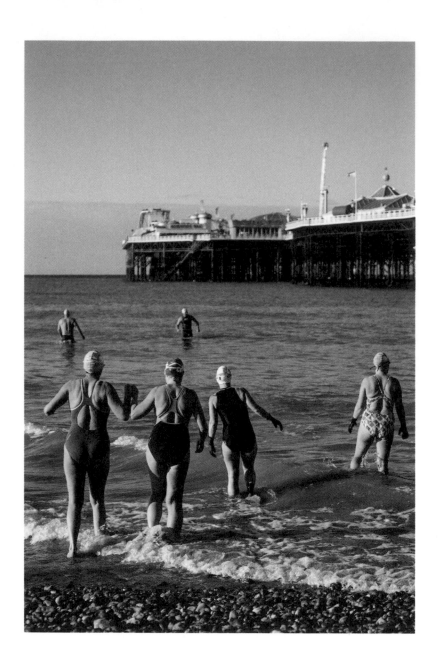

44 Bathe

British bathing

British bathing needs sprang from the practical and communal demand for cleanliness.

In ancient times, public bathing included saunas, massages and relaxation therapies comparable to today's spas. In the Middle Ages most people didn't have access to private bathing facilities. Wells and the streams of monasteries provided clean water, and bathhouses emerged in many towns around Britain. Most types of 'public' baths in the Middle Ages were, in fact, restricted to certain members of the public and entrance depended on things like affordability, gender or religious persuasion. In the 14th century, Edward III installed a bathroom in the Palace of Westminster, while mere mortals made do with wooden tubs in their bedrooms. In the 16th century, when bathrooms were still very rare, Henry VIII had a bathroom put in Hampton Court Palace with a simple boiler for hot water. But it wasn't until the mid-19th century that middle-class homes began to have their own bathrooms. By the mid-19th century, the English urbanised middle classes had started to liken cleanliness with the majority of other Victorian concepts, including Christianity, respectability and social standing. Cleanliness was king!

INTRODUCTION

Wild bathing: Hidden dips in rivers, lakes and waterfalls

Wild bathing can be a freeing feeling like no other and has been practised since the beginnings of time: Stepping into clear, cool waters on a baking hot summer's day, bringing with it a sense of freedom, adventure and fun and lazing on the grass nearby to dry out afterwards. Diving into icy, gin-clear water, or a bathwater-warm jungle cenote (sinkhole) with every shade of rippling blue and green has to be the ultimate in healing and detoxing: Just you, your wet suit, swimming costume or birthday suit, and the water. Both exhilarating and energising, it brings us up close and personal with Mother Nature and pares life back to its purest elements of water, air and earth.

Relax in buoyant sea water, surrounded by crabs and cliffs; luxuriate in the silky softness of river waters and gently float downstream while gazing at clouds or delight in the gentle pleasure of relaxing in tranquil lakes, ponds and tarns. These bathing experiences are more curative than ever before and an antidote to our modern-day, technology-filled lives, reconnecting us with nature and bringing peace and stillness with them. This is perhaps why the current wild swimming movement has never been stronger.

There are many sublime natural locations around the globe for wild swimming. Many are in tropical countries – Central and South America, with their largely untouched, ancient jungle landscapes, are rich in lagoons and ancient cave pools. At Bacalar in Mexico, a lagoon of seven colours reveals itself as you swim to the middle, changing from pastel blue to deep cobalt. These feel like a secret underworld, where you lose all sense of time, and are so dramatic that they hosted the 2014 Red Bull Cliff Diving World Series.

In Britain there are popular wild swimming spots too. From Kenwood Ladies' Pond in Hampstead, North London, to the Strait of Corryvreckan in Scotland, where you can find one of the world's biggest and most dramatic whirlpools. Time your dash across it badly, when the whirlpool is active, and you could end up badly injured, if not killed, so much so that the 1km swim can only be done with supervision. On the Isle of Skye, the romantically named Fairy Pools, at the foot of the Black Cuillin, are a series of crystal-clear blue pools.

There is truly an almost animalistic wildness (some might say madness!) about this nature of swimming. For many it becomes a lifestyle choice, as they push themselves to try a bucket list of dips – the colder the better – many of which are in remote locations and feature sub-zero temperatures. The gasp-inducing cold of the water creates a natural high for the body and mind. Reputed to even trigger a release of happy hormones, it is something that can easily become addictive, thrilling and death defying! To others who opt for the tamer waters – simply, nature's public pool – it is a place to feel alive again, and a place free of chlorine, rules and ceilings!

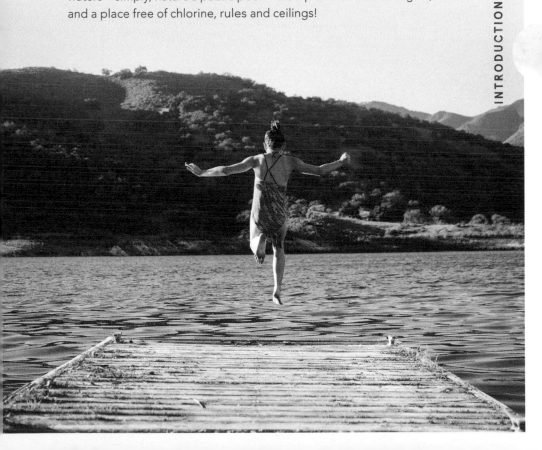

Purify

'Water is life, and clean
water means health'

[AUDREY HEPBURN]

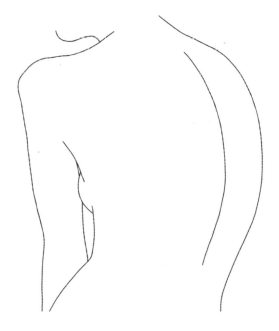

51 Bathe

Regularly cleansing and purifying our bodies is essential for good health, and bathing can be transformed into a healing act.

Did you know that our skin – which is our largest organ – is sometimes called the third kidney, due to the role it plays in detoxing our bodies? Detoxification is the body's way of removing and metabolising dangerous compounds. Warm water stimulates detoxification through the skin, kidneys, liver and colon by encouraging lymphatic flow, boosting circulation and encouraging sweating. Bathing has always helped us to do this very easily and with very little expense. You get similar benefits to those gained in a high-end spa but at a fraction of the cost and in the comfort of your own home too.

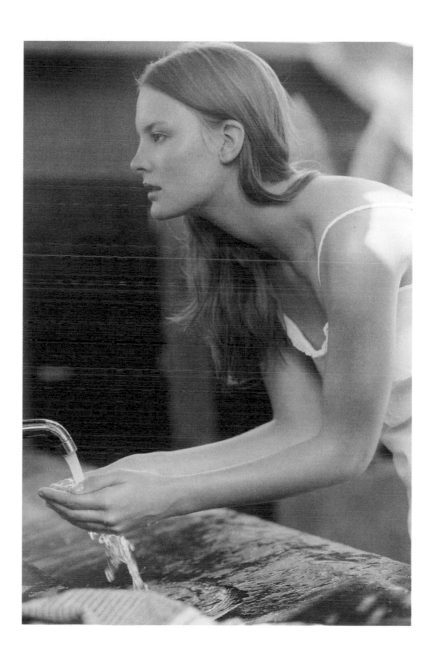

53 Bathe

Power baths

When you hear the call of your bathtub, you'd be wise to listen. Even the ancient Romans knew that everything could be cured with a soak. Modern maladies can be remedied in the tub too if you immerse yourself in a bath brimming with the best ingredients to support internal and external cleansing. Powerful homemade recipes can revive mind and body turning a simple steep into a power bath!

BENEFITS OF SALTS, MUDS AND OILS FOR THE SKIN

Bathing ingredients can be chosen to target specific ailments, including many skin problems and other conditions or injuries, such as muscle pain. Salts, muds and oils are easy to use, affordable and safe for almost everyone.

SALTS

The benefits of bathing salts are wide-ranging and can boost our bodies from the inside out. In their natural form, they contain many nutrients and minerals, including magnesium, potassium, sodium and calcium. When bathing, warm water opens our pores, allowing these minerals to be absorbed, purifying and cleansing the skin and enhancing its texture and radiance. This also draws out pollution, impurities, toxins and dirt, and even calms the nervous system.

All of these minerals have far-reaching advantages – they are like superfoods for the skin. As well as aiding detoxification, the minerals in salts have different benefits: Magnesium raises serotonin levels, which eases stress; it also helps mitigate inflammation and muscular soreness and keeps blood pressure in check; calcium boosts circulation, strengthens bones and nails and can help to stave off diseases like osteoporosis; potassium energises and balances skin moisture, while sodium balances lymphatic fluid and consequently the immune system.

Popular salts include Epsom salts, (also known as magnesium sulfate) Dead Sea salts and Himalayan salts, all of which are wonderful additions to a bath.

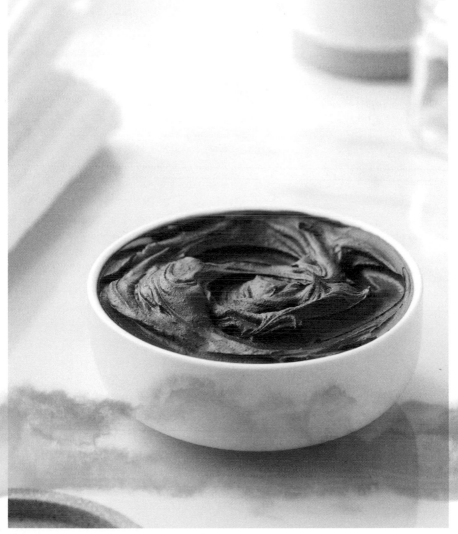

MUDS

It might seem counter-intuitive to bathe in mud, but for thousands of years, people have believed in the health benefits of mud, and in ancient times, muds were considered a cure for almost any ailment. Like salts, muds and other clays and peats are rich in minerals such as magnesium, potassium and sodium, nourishing the skin and body. With an alkaline pH and negative ionic charge, muds also have a gentle pulling action, which shrinks pores, exfoliates and detoxifies. This promotes a more youthful complexion, hence the popularity of mud masks.

Mud from hot springs, volcanoes and marine sediments contains the highest amount of minerals, and mud from the Dead Sea, the deepest and most saline lake on earth, is said to contain high concentrations of magnesium, phosphates, bromides and other minerals. Scientific studies have shown that Dead Sea mud is particularly beneficial for skin conditions like psoriasis, eczema and acne and has also proven useful in the treatment of rheumatologic diseases, including arthritis.

OILS

When mixed with water, oil has the ability to penetrate deep into the skin and provides rejuvenation. This helps to soften and nourish the skin and has been scientifically proven to reduce signs of dryness and improve some skin conditions.

Most bath oils use a base oil, scented with an essential oil, and this is one of the easiest ways to implement aromatherapy and its benefits. Natural oils are recommended by experts for both their purity and efficacy. These oils are made using medicinal plants, flowers, herbs, roots and trees, which have proven and powerful effects on the body. From supporting the immune system, treating respiratory issues and soothing inflammation, through to promoting a sense of well-being, relaxing and calming the mind and inducing sleep, the power of aromatherapy is far-reaching.

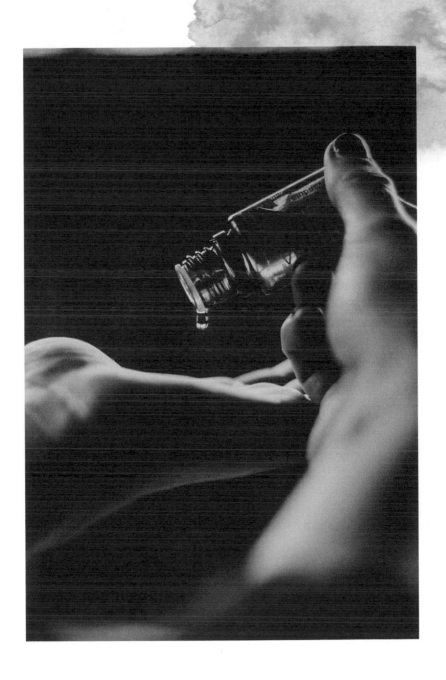

FOUR DETOXING BATH RECIPES
FOR IMPROVED HEALTH

There are few things as relaxing as a detox bath. A good detox bath will restore balance, fight illness, boost the body's natural detoxifying process, improve circulation, soothe muscles and create a sense of mental clarity too. The detoxifying recipes can make you a little tired as the body is triggered into detoxifying, so go slow afterwards and if time allows, wrap up in a warm towel.

In the pink

Himalayan pink salt is rich in essential minerals and trace elements and widely used in the cosmetic, culinary and medical fields. This beautiful, hand-mined salt is extracted from the Himalayan mountains and is known to be the purest one on earth. It is accompanied by a plethora of health and healing properties, including boosting circulation and balancing the moisture of the skin. Vibrant grapefruit oil acts as a gentle stimulant to the lymphatic system, aiding the body's natural toxin elimination process, and it also tones skin and soothes nerves. Warming and comforting ginger is a stimulating essential oil that aids circulation, enhancing the body's natural healing process.

120g/½ cup Himalayan pink salt
120g/½ cup Epsom salt
1 tsp bicarbonate of soda
    (baking soda)
2 drops of grapefruit oil
2 drops of ginger oil

Pour all of the ingredients into the tub as the warm water starts to fill the bath. Soak for up to 30 minutes.

PURIFY

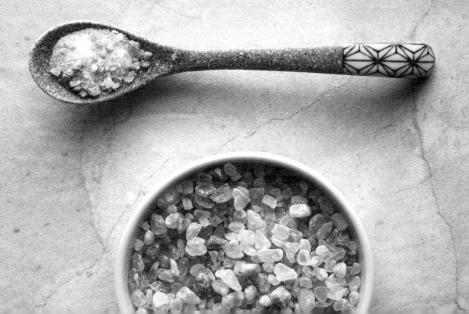

Bring the beach to your bath

The countless vitamins, minerals and nutrients in the salts and seaweed help relieve stress, aches and pains, encourage the body to expel toxins, help induce sleep and even help to balance hormones. Quality seaweed powder is brimming with vitamin C, which boosts collagen production and skin elasticity; potassium, which is needed for proper hydration of the body, including the skin; and iron, which promotes circulation of blood throughout the body and provides the skin with abundant oxygen-rich blood, which makes it healthy and supple. Additionally, it is packed with choline, an essential micronutrient which soothes skin irritation and revitalises mature skin. A top-to-toe toning tonic!

60g/¼ cup Epsom salts
60g/¼ cup Dead Sea salt
120g/½ cup seaweed powder
For an added sensory boost
   (and to help distract from
   the pungent sea smell!),
   add 7–10 drops of one
   of the following essential
   oils: juniper berry, lavender,
   sandalwood or patchouli

Combine the salts and seaweed powder in a container, then stir into a hot bath. Amp up your bath with no more than 10 drops in total of essential oils. Soak for 20 – 30 minutes.

PURIFY

'Quality seaweed powder is brimming with vitamin C, which boosts collagen production and skin elasticity'

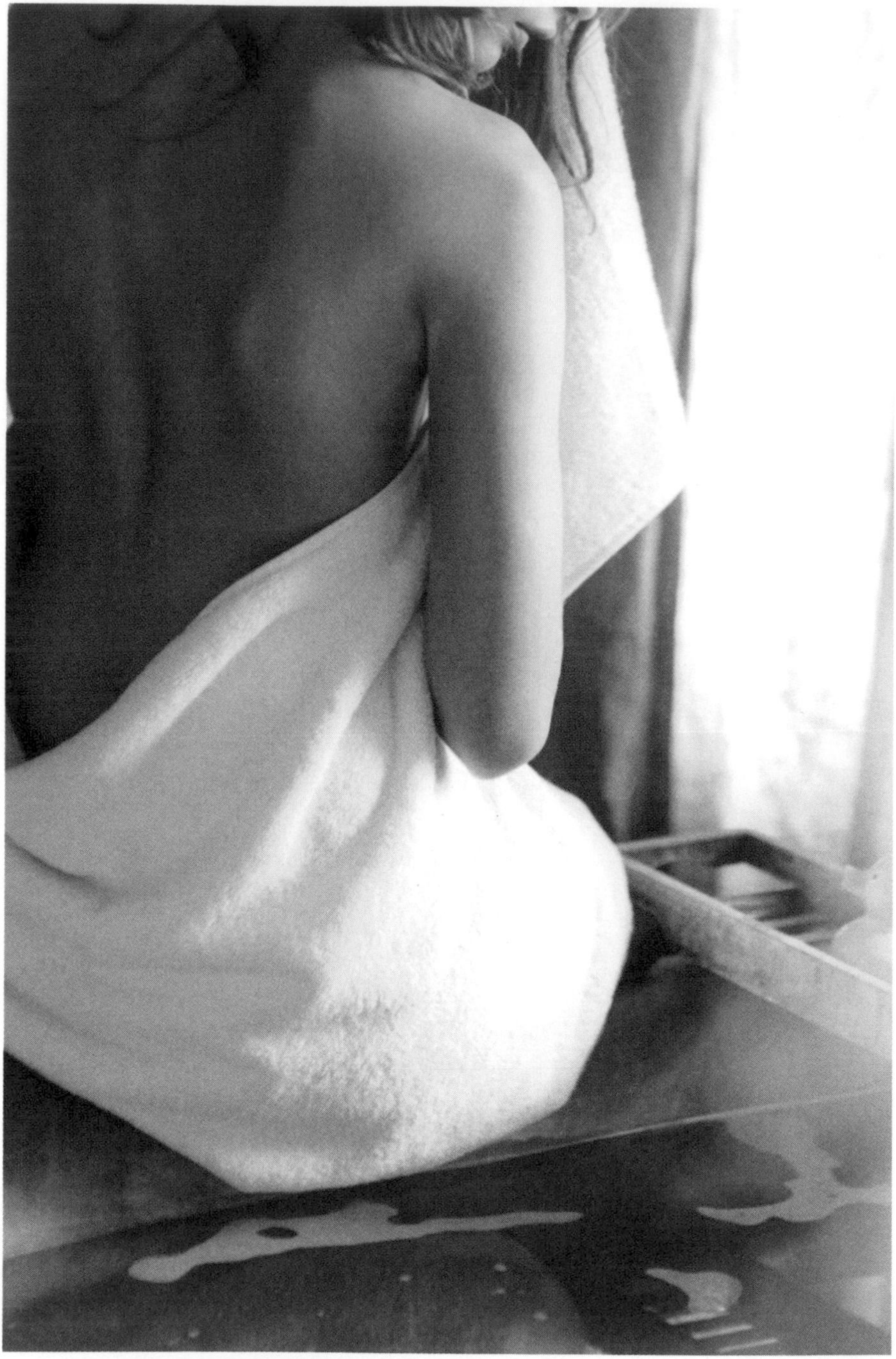

Cleansing and calming
salts and clay combo

Epsom salts are an excellent source of magnesium, a miracle mineral that aids sleep and calms the nervous system. Bentonite clay pulls toxins from the skin and gently exfoliates, and both lavender and frankincense essential oils help create tranquillity, relax the mind and soothe anxiety. Most high-grade natural sodium bentonite is produced in the western United States in an area between the Black Hills of South Dakota and the Bighorn Basin of Wyoming.

120g/½ cup Epsom salts
120g/½ cup bentonite clay
3 drops of French lavender
  essential oil
3 drops of frankincense
  essential oil

Combine the salt, clay and oils in a hot bath. Then sit in the detox concoction for 25–30 minutes.

PURIFY

Purifying fresh herbs and baking soda soak

Baking soda, or bicarbonate of soda as it is known in the UK, is a salt composed of sodium ions and bicarbonate ions and is a great detoxifier and skin softener. Look for the aluminium-free version to add to your bath. Parsley will soothe inflammation and tone skin, mint is known to aid healing, and the addition of rosemary will leave you relaxed and calm.

2 tbsp Epsom salts or sea salt
1 tsp bicarbonate of soda
(baking soda)
1 tsp extra virgin olive oil
A generous bunch of bruised
parsley, rosemary and mint
in a tied muslin cloth or
cheesecloth to keep the
bath clean

Add all the ingredients to warm bathwater and enjoy.

PURIFY

NOTES

Use an eco or natural bath cleaner
so that you are not soaking in the residue
of a chemical cleaning product

Have a little bucket with a bath sponge
or cloth to ensure easy cleaning afterwards
– oil, seaweeds and clay need to be
cleaned off straight away to avoid
that unappealing tide mark.

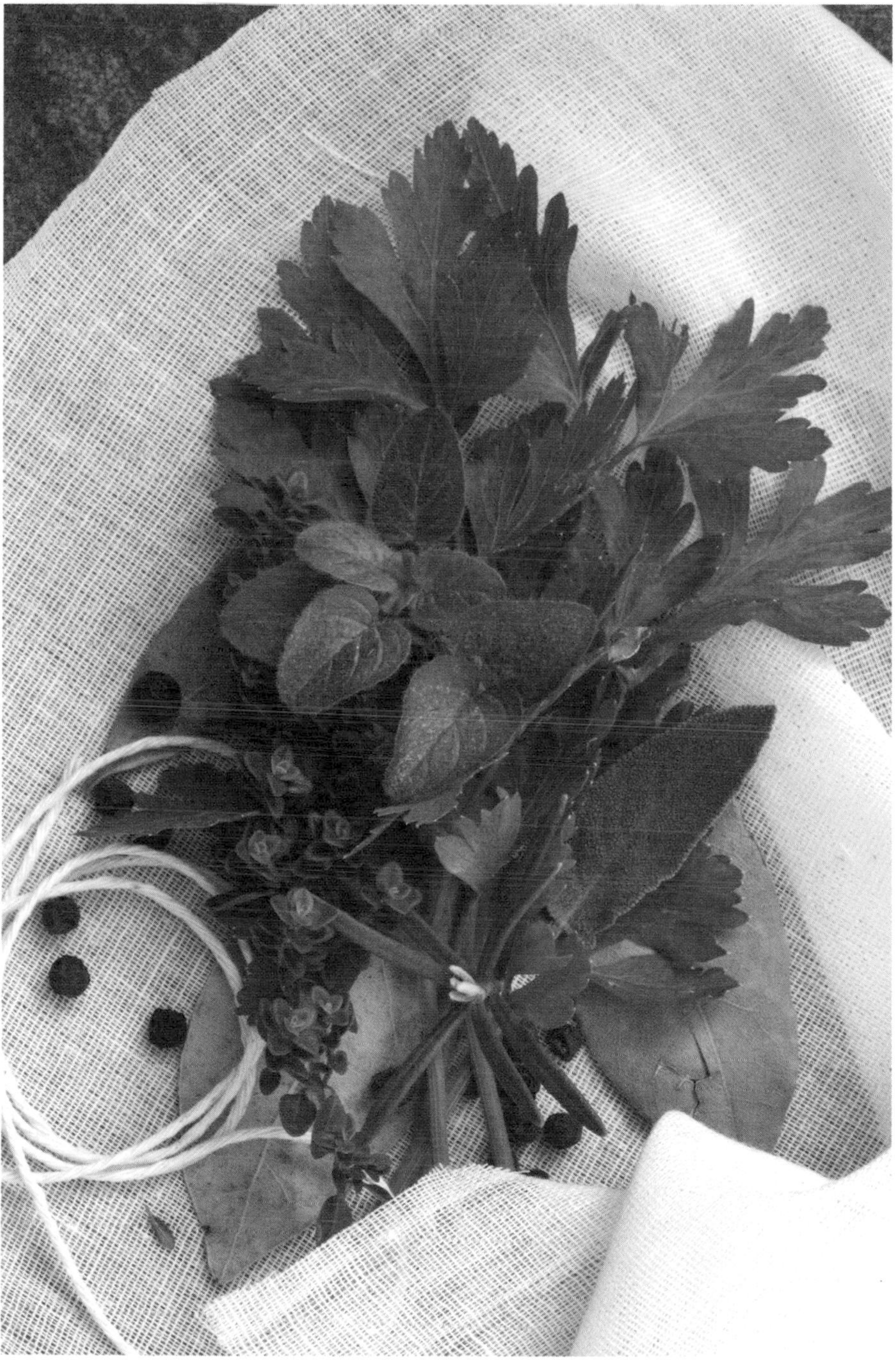

FIVE RESTORATIVE RECIPES
FOR BODY AND MIND

Bath recipes should be considered and curated in the same way as we do food recipes for they are the wellness worlds equivalent of a marinade – a seasoned liquid often using salt, herb, spices and oils to steep foods in before cooking. Like a meal, a bath with the perfect ingredients can change the mood, improve health, nourish and promote feelings of happiness and being comforted. Essential oils have been used for their powerful medicinal and spiritual health purposes for centuries and incorporating the right essential oils and other accompaniments depending on your emotional and physical needs and their specific health promoting properties, can seriously turbo-charge your time in the tub.

Pregnant women or people with certain health conditions like heart conditions and high blood pressure should consult with their doctor before use.

The Energiser

for increased vitality and energy

When you're wired on caffeine but still feel exhausted, it's time to look for another solution. This bath is not just reserved for evening unwinding; it's an effective pick-me-up, ideal for taking in the morning too, and the almond oil will ensure the oils mix effectively and stay on your skin, giving the added bonus of skin conditioning. Grapefruit oil has a fresh and zesty smell that will awaken your senses and draw out impurities, leaving you feeling physically lighter. Run your bath to a warm temperature, or run it slightly cooler if you want to be even more refreshed.

60ml/¼ cup of almond oil (you can also use olive oil or coconut oil)
240g/1¼ cup granulated sugar
10 drops of grapefruit essential oil

Add the almond oil to the sugar until you get the consistency that you like, before adding the grapefruit essential oil. Mix thoroughly and put into an airtight container. This can be kept for up to three months, though use generously, so it will probably last less time. Always use a clean spoon to extract the scrub, so it is not contaminated with bacteria.

When you bathe, mindfully rub the scrub on your body with a little water. Bathe and then rinse with warm water (especially if your water temperature is cooler) to remove excess oils. This will exfoliate your skin and leave it soft, smooth and zinging with freshness.

PURIFY

The Reviver
for aching muscles

Doing workouts, feeling stressed and poor posture can all leave us with sore and achy muscles that feel tender and swollen. This bath recipe will hit all your sore spots. Juniper is known for its antiseptic and soothing properties, marjoram oil helps to relieve muscle cramps and tension, while arnica reduces pain and inflammation.

5 drops of marjoram oil
5 drops of arnica oil
5 drops of juniper oil
2 tbsp milk

Run the water hot. Mix the oils with milk to ensure even distribution. Soak for 20 minutes to allow the oils to penetrate.

The Upper
for low mood

If you are feeling drained and anxious, sad or generally run down, the right bath can help. Orange essential oil is a wonderful mood lifter. The oil is extracted from the peel of oranges and contains many antidepressant properties and has been scientifically proven to help reduce heart rate and cortisol levels.

500ml/2 cups coconut oil
250g/1 cup Epsom salts
5 drops of orange oil

Run your bath but don't step in right away. Splash your body first with water to dampen your skin before rubbing this orangey body scrub head to toe in circular motions. Soak for at least 15 minutes so that the oils have time to take effect.

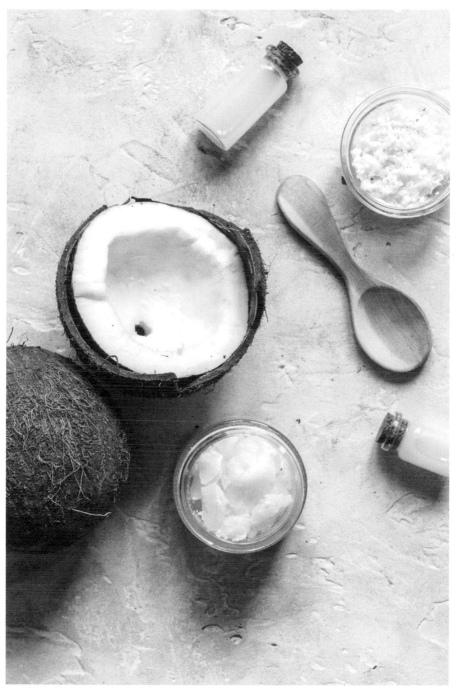

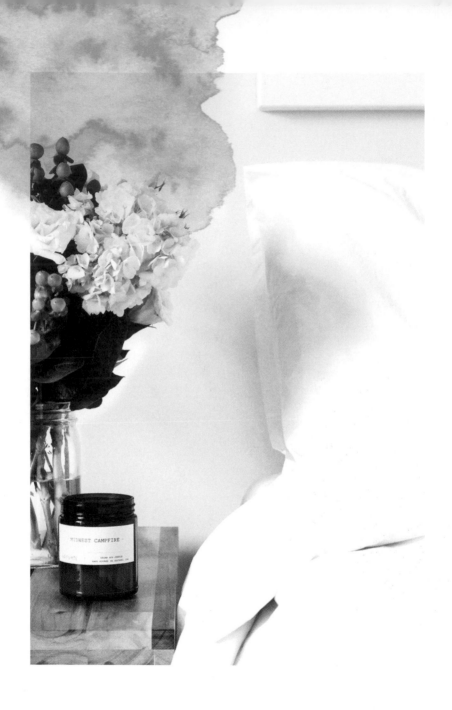

PURIFY

MIDWEST CAMPFIRE

The Sleep Inducer
for deep and restful shut-eye

Lavender is the scent of choice for sleep. The Romans added it to their bathwater (the word comes from the Latin word 'lavare', which means 'to wash'). Lavender is used in many sleep blends. Look out for French high-altitude lavender oil because it contains higher natural linalyl acetate (ester) levels, so its properties are enhanced. Cedarwood is also known for its comforting, grounding and warm scent. This oil supports the healthy function of the pineal gland, which releases melotonin, the body's natural sleep hormone.

5 drops of high-altitude
   lavender oil
3 drops of cedarwood oil
2 tbsp milk

Add the oils to the milk before pouring into a hot bath. Soak for 20 minutes and feel the slumber-inducing effects take place.

PURIFY

The Aphrodisiac

for romance

It's hard to find a more romantic oil than rose. It is calming, reduces anxiety and is traditionally used as an aphrodisiac because it is said to stir desire and enhance self-esteem and confidence. Men might like to use clary sage oil because it has a balmy and earthy scent and is both deeply relaxing and a powerful aphrodisiac. Milk leaves the skin soft and smooth and is a great carrier for oils.

10 tbsp rose petals
10 drops of rose essential oil/
    clary sage oil
300g/4 cups milk powder

PURIFY

Place the rose petals in a large bowl or measuring jug and sprinkle with the essential oil – not only do they look pretty but they give the oil something to adhere to. Mix with a spoon so they are well covered. Add in the milk powder and stir well until the rose petals are evenly distributed; use your hands, if it is easier. Sprinkle a teacupful over your warm bathwater once it's finished running and stir in – the smell is amazing! Soak for at least ten minutes to enjoy the skin-softening benefits.

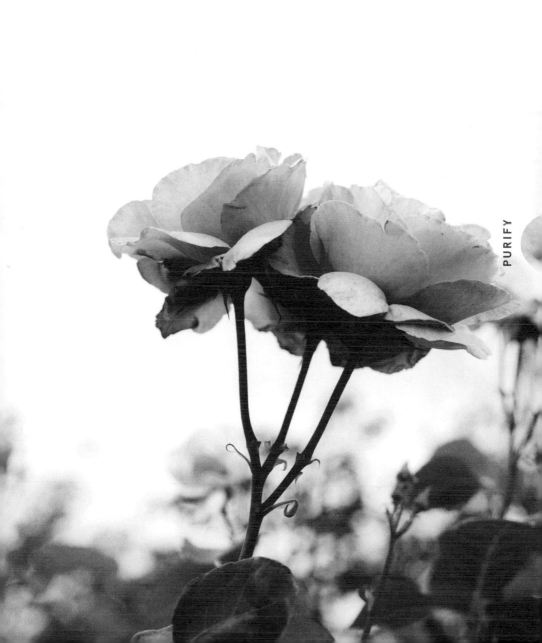

PURIFY

The simple beauty
of Japanese onsen

Onsen bathing is a beloved and important part of Japanese culture and permeates society, transcending social, economic, generational and geographical barriers. An onsen ('hot water spring') is a natural hot spring bath and soaking in these baths is known as 'toji' (hot spring cure). There are 3,000 hot springs, which power spa resorts across the country and as an island nation poised atop active volcanoes, every region of the country has its fair share.

Official onsen are ones that contain 19 naturally occurring chemical elements and the water must emerge out of the ground at 25°C or hotter. The water is rich in sulphur and sodium chloride, which is thought to heal aches and pains, as well as help with conditions such as hypertension and diabetes. All onsen are simple, clean spaces, brimming with elegance and taste. Most onsen are single-sex, but some onsen, known as 'konyoku', are mixed baths, where men and women can bathe together.

Many onsen are resplendent in marble, glass and tiles in huge, bustling cities, while others are more low-key affairs and set outside. Soaking in a hot spring, amongst the natural scenery of the surrounding mountains and forests gives a sense of harmony, the shift of the seasons and becoming one with the natural world, and enhances the joy of the wonders of nature, such as snow and cherry blossom. Many hot springs are located near some of Japan's most picturesque spots.

Rotenburo are open-air baths and sometimes include hot waterfalls and other natural features. Bathers can gaze up at the spectacular Mount Fuji, rising from the sweeping blue Sea of Japan; they can surround themselves with an autumnal display of fiery red and orange leaves or become bewitched by the delicate pink cherry blooms that emerge during the spring months. Many bathers indulge in one of the nation's favourite pastimes – hanami – which translated means 'looking at flowers'.

Onsen baths can be beautiful objects in themselves, made from materials like granite, marble and wood to imbue a sense of ambience. One of the best places to experience an onsen is through a ryokan, a traditional inn, which are built on or near the site of the source of the onsen. These often feature Japanese-style wooden architecture and Zen gardens. Guests sleep in traditional rooms, furnished with futons, low tables and floor cushions on 'tatami' bamboo mats. Some onsen ryokan have become dedicated Japanese cultural heritage sites, where you can sense, hear and feel the ambience of days gone by.

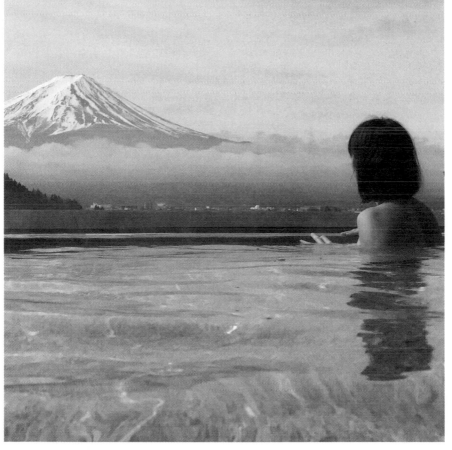

PURIFY

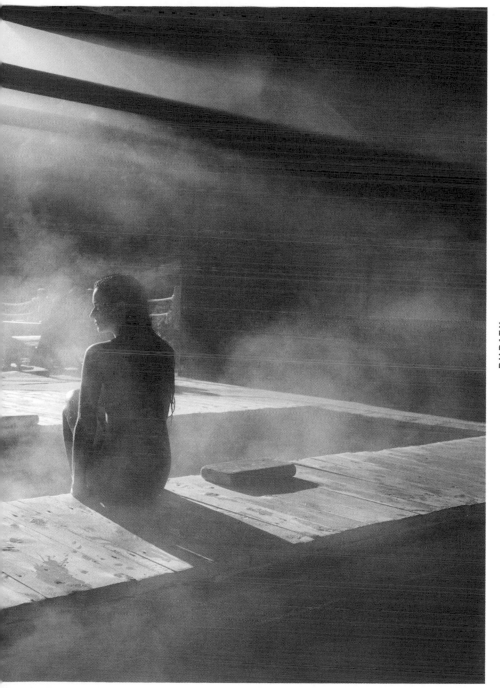

PURIFY

JAPANESE ETIQUETTE:
HOW TO ONSEN

Like every country, Japan has many unwritten rules about etiquette. The Japanese bathing ritual is simple, subtle and graceful.

Wash carefully before you enter the water: This is probably the most important rule of Japanese bathing. In Japanese culture, bathing is for cleansing and purifying the body first, then for relaxation. Even in the privacy of their own homes, the Japanese always shower before taking a bath. Most Japanese onsen have a separate showering area away from the water, with small stools to sit on. In very simple baths, bathers are expected to crouch by the edge of the bath and scoop the water to rinse themselves before hopping in.

No shoes allowed: Many onsen have traditional tatami mat flooring. It is customary to remove your shoes before stepping into the onsen area.

Birthday suits only: The Japanese are so accustomed to public bathing that being naked is second nature. Swimsuits are typically not permitted.

Use two towels: In all onsen, bathers are provided with a large towel and a smaller one. The large one is left in the changing area, while the smaller one is taken in for washing; some people take them into the baths, but they must not get in the water. Many people wear them on their heads!

Tie long hair up: People with long hair are expected to tie it up or wrap it in a small towel, even if it has just been washed, for hygiene reasons.

Tattoos are strictly forbidden: The reason for this is because they are associated with Yakuza, the Japanese mafia. This means that tattoos are banned from onsen and sento (Japanese bathing houses where the water is heated by boilers) completely.

Keep the noise down! Most onsen are sociable places where people chat and commune, but noisy or boisterous behaviour is not accepted.

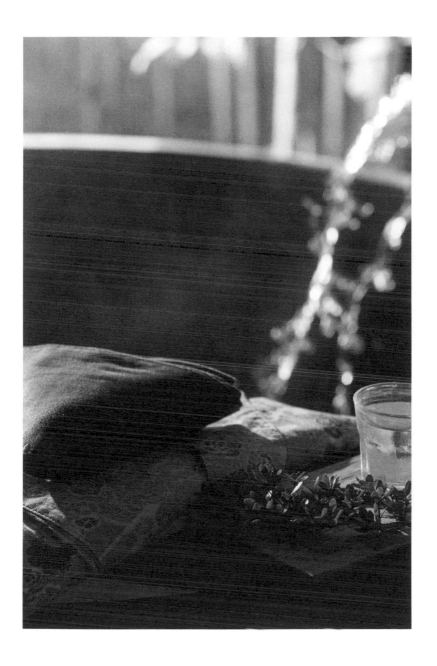

79 Bathe

Sentos vs onsen

There are obvious similarities between onsen and sentos: both are communal bathhouses where people go to soak their hot, tired bodies and socialise with friends and neighbours, and both have a clear etiquette for visitors to follow. The single most important difference is that onsen are filled with natural water from hot springs, while sentos run on heated tap water, though some sentos add infusions and minerals to the water.

Sentos are neighbourhood bathhouses, which provide a unique atmosphere and a place to meet with the locals and wash your troubles away. In the post-war era, few people had access to their own private baths because countless homes were damaged or destroyed, so many people routinely bathed in their local sento. Now, every home has a bathtub and the numbers of sentos are dwindling. However, they are still a common sight in many older residential areas, dotted within old shopping districts or along streets that are lined with older houses. Here are places where you will see old men scrub each others' backs, visitors say goodnight to everyone as they leave and old ladies exfoliate their faces fiercely.

In some areas of Japan there are super-sentos, where all the benefits of countryside hot spring resorts are brought into towns. Here, visitors will find state-of-the-art bathing equipment, restaurants, gyms, reading rooms, saunas and massage facilities.

PURIFY

'The single most important difference is that onsen are filled with natural water from hot springs, while sentos run on heated tap water, though some sentos add infusions and minerals to the water'

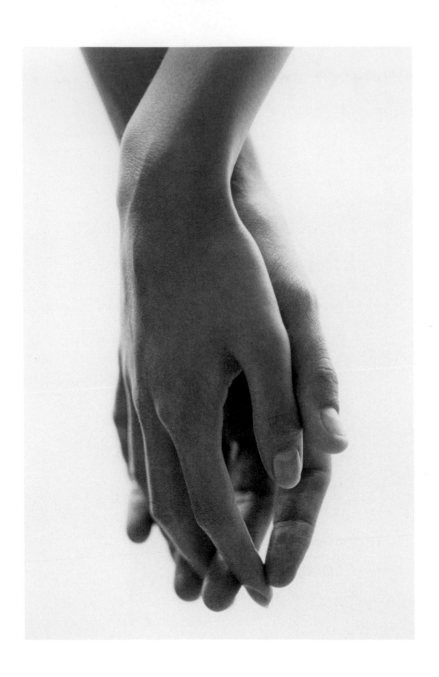

82   Bathe

What is 'skinship'?

In Japan and South Korea, the term 'skinship' is used to describe non-sexual touching and an intimacy between family or friends. Co-bathing is widely considered the ultimate scenario in skinship. This is an important and valued form of intimacy because bathing naked symbolises the removal of social trappings and barriers that separate us. Hierarchy and status are not apparent or important when naked. This fosters closeness and promotes bonding, friendship and equality.

PURIFY

'...bathing
naked symbolises
the removal of
social trappings
and barriers that
separate us'

PURIFY

It's not just humans who love onsen!

The old adage 'monkey see, monkey do' is apt in this case. While the Japanese have been bathing in onsen for centuries, more recently the onsen has been adopted by another population: the wild macaques of Nagano, otherwise known as Japan's 'snow monkeys'. During the winter, the Jigokudani Monkey Park, at the base of the Shiga Kogen region, is a real paradise for monkeys, who use their own private streaming hot springs to keep themselves warm. Their behaviour is surprisingly similar to that of humans; while the adult monkeys mainly use the spring for relaxation purposes, with their heads back and their eyes closed, the young macaques treat it as a social occasion, grooming each other and playing.

HOW TO BATHE JAPANESE-STYLE

The traditional Japanese bathing ritual has been perfected over centuries and for many, it is a meditative practice. It is easy to incorporate some of the essential elements of Japanese bathing into your own routine.

Often performed in the evening, Japanese bathing is done in two stages: first, cleansing the body, then it is equally important to relax and let the day's troubles float away.

Set the tone: Dim the lights or light candles. Make sure the bathroom is clear of clutter and a calm place to be. Take a few minutes to appreciate the moment.

Prepare the bath: Fill your bathtub ahead of time. Clear, hot water is fine; a temperature of 36 to 38°C is about right. Use cooler water if it is hot outside.

Cleanse the body: Shower your body first and wash carefully with your choice of soap or cleanser and water, including your hair, if you wish. The Japanese hate the idea of bathing in dirty bathwater. They don't mess around when it comes to scrubbing themselves down, cleansing from head to toe, using a washcloth held at either end.

Immerse yourself: When you have scrubbed yourself, ease into the bath slowly, allowing your body to adjust to the temperature. Splash some water over your shoulders and chest.

Soak: Relax in the bath for pure enjoyment. This is the time to be present and nurture yourself, reflect on your day and take advantage of the solitude. Let your muscles unwind and slow your breathing. Try to relax for at least 20 minutes.

Exit the bath: Take a moment to relax and ground yourself as you get out of the bath. Take a few deep breaths. Some people like to rinse in the shower with cooler water before wrapping themselves in a clean, cotton robe.

The moment afterwards: 'Yuagari' translates as 'the moment after the bath'. This is the perfect time to do nothing or relax in whatever way you please: take a nap, listen to music, sip some tea, or read a book.

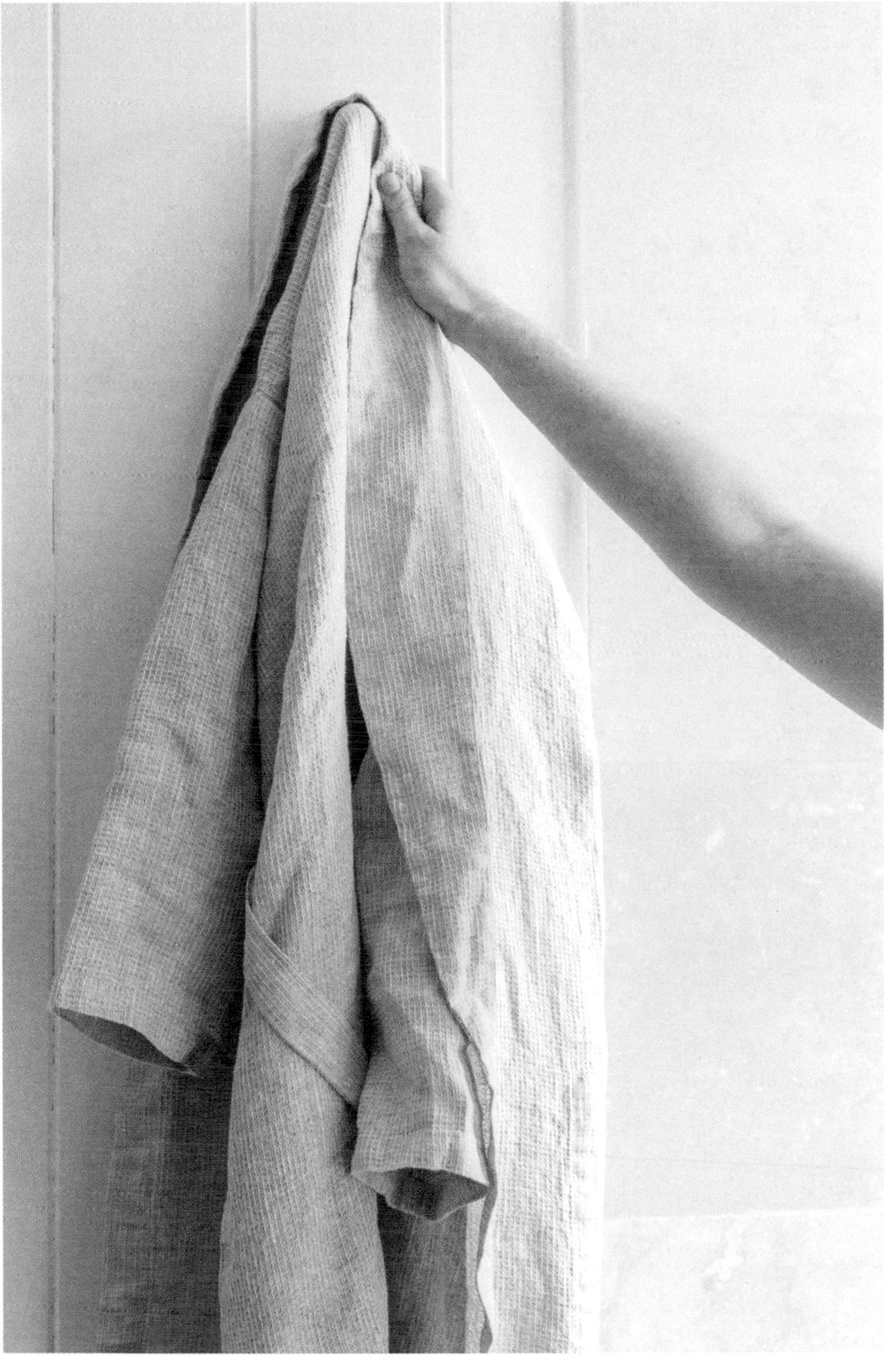

Excerpt from Yasunari Kawabata's *Snow Country*

In *Snow Country*, Nobel Prize-winning author Yasunari Kawabata tells the powerful tale of a fleeting and doomed love affair between wealthy Tokyo dilettante Shimamura and a lowly, provincial geisha girl. Set within a hot spring town in Niigata province on the west coast of Japan, the story is told in lyrical and simple prose and many things are conveyed indirectly. This part of the novel tells of the night when Shimamura and the geisha girl – who he later learns is called Komako – go to the bath before spending the night together.

It was a stern night landscape. The sound of the freezing of snow over the land seemed to roar deep into the earth. There was no moon. The stars, almost too many of them to be true, came forward so brightly that it was as if they were falling with the swiftness of the void. As the stars came nearer, the sky retreated deeper and deeper into the night colour. The layers of the Border Range, indistinguishable one from another, cast their heaviness at the skirt of the starry sky in a blackness grave and sombre enough to communicate their mass. The whole of the night scene came together in a clear, tranquil harmony.

As she sensed Shimamura's approach, the woman fell over with her breast against the railing. There was no hint of weakness in the pose. Rather, against the night, it was the strongest and most stubborn she could have taken. So we have to go through this again, thought Shimamura.

Black though the mountains were, they seemed at that moment brilliant with the colour of the snow. They seemed to him somehow transparent, somehow lonely. The harmony between sky and mountains was lost.

Shimamura put his hand to the woman's throat. 'You'll catch cold. See how cold it is.' He tried to pull her back, but she clung to the railing.

'I'm going home.' Her voice was choked.

'Go home, then.'

'Let me stay like this a little longer.'

'I'm going down for a bath.'

'No, stay here with me.'

'If you close the window.'

'Let me stay here like this a little longer.'

Half the village was hidden behind the cedars of the shrine grove. The light in the railway station, not ten minutes away by taxi, flickered on and off as if crackling in the cold.

The woman's hair, the glass of the window, the sleeve of his kimono – everything he touched was cold in a way Shimamura had never known before.

Even the straw mats under his feet seemed cold. He started down to the bath.

'Wait, I'll go with you.' The woman followed meekly.

As she was rearranging the clothes he had thrown to the floor outside the bath, another guest, a man, came in. The woman crouched low in front of Shimamura and hid her face.

'Excuse me.' The other guests started to back away.

'No, please,' Shimamura said quickly. 'We'll go next door.'

He scooped up his clothes and stepped over to the women's bath. The woman followed as if they were married. Shimamura plunged into the bath without looking back at her. He felt a high laugh mount on his lips now that he knew she was with him. He put his face to the hot water tap and noisily rinsed his mouth.

PURIFY

A SIMPLE BATHTIME BREATHING EXERCISE TO PURIFY THE MIND AND RELAX THE NERVOUS SYSTEM

The 4-7-8 breathing exercise is a natural tranquiliser for the nervous system and while it feels subtle when you first try it, it gains in power and effect with repetition and practice. You can do it in any position, but sitting in the bath with your back straight is preferable while learning the exercise because sitting up straight helps with focus and encourages your lungs to fill and empty.

Place the tip of your tongue against the ridge of tissue just behind your front top teeth for the whole exercise. You will be exhaling through your mouth around your tongue; try pursing your lips slightly if this helps.

Take a normal breath and exhale completely through your mouth, making a whooshing sound.

Close your mouth and inhale quietly through your nose to a count of four.

Hold your breath for a count of seven.

Exhale completely through your mouth, making a whoosh sound to a count of eight.

This is one round. Repeat the cycle three more times for a total of four rounds.

Your exhalations should take twice as long as inhalations and the ratio of 4-7-8 is important. If you have trouble holding your breath, speed the exercise up, but keep to the ratio of 4-7-8 and with practice you can slow it all down and get used to inhaling and exhaling more deeply. Try to do it at least twice a day and always when bathing. You cannot do it too frequently but don't take more than four breaths at one time for the first three to four weeks of practising. Then, if you like, you can extend it to eight rounds.

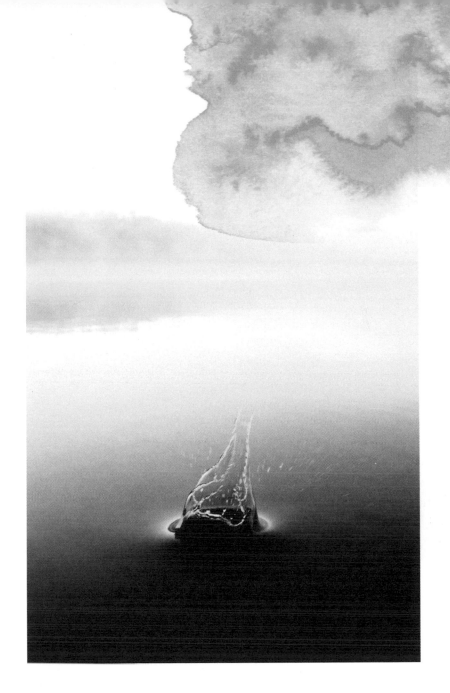

91   Bathe

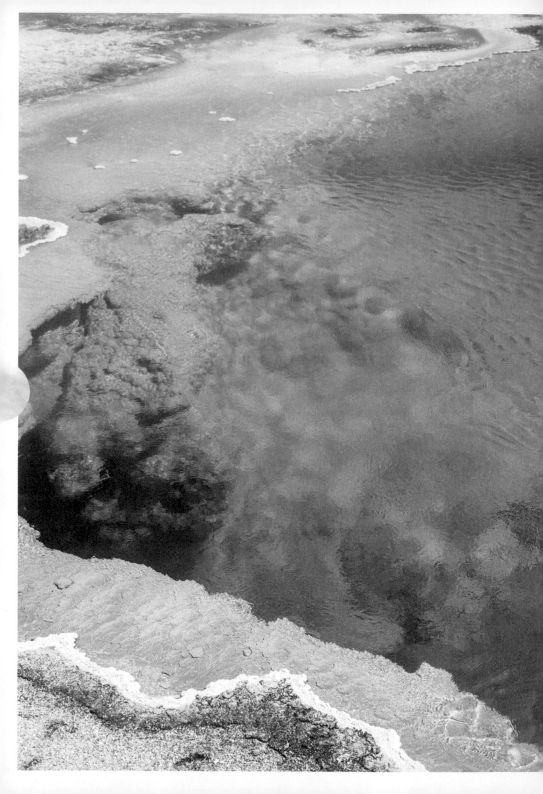

Five of the best natural spas for a soak

When you are deciding where next to go on your travels, resorts with natural hot springs are dotted all over the globe. From remote mountainside villages to busy city centres, natural spas are wondrous phenomena offering self-care and pampering. Here are just a handful to inspire your next trip.

DEAD SEA, JORDAN AND ISRAEL

At 400m below sea level and at the lowest point on earth, the climate makes the Dead Sea unique. This is one of the safest places to sunbathe because harmful ultraviolet rays are filtered. Mineral-rich mud and the opportunity to bathe in the saltiest sea in the world, attracts thousands of people each year seeking its health-giving properties. The natural environment is said not only to purify the skin, but aids everything from skin conditions to joint pain, respiratory issues and heart problems.

THERMAE BATH SPA, BATH

The hot springs of Bath, from which the city derives its name, offer mineral-rich waters for bathing. This is Britain's only original and natural thermal spa and has been enjoyed by everyone from the Celts to the Saxons. The buildings have been restored, using the existing Georgian buildings and contemporary design features. With delightfully warm waters containing 42 different minerals, visitors can enjoy a series of different pools, including the open-air rooftop pool, with stunning views across the honey-coloured city.

PURIFY

BLUE LAGOON, ICELAND

Nestled in one of Iceland's black lava fields, mineral-rich hot water from beneath the earth's surface fills a spectacular lagoon with turquoise-blue waters. It is one of the most visited spots in Iceland. The bright blue (sometimes green-tinged) colour comes from the silica in the water and the way it reflects sunlight. A couple of luxurious health spas have been developed here, with a host of amenities. The geothermal waters are said to tighten, exfoliate and rejuvenate the skin and offer other health benefits too, such as helping with respiratory problems, including asthma, and boosting circulation. Tubs of white, geothermal mud are available to guests so they can apply their own face masks.

TERMAS BAÑOS DE PURITAMA, CHILE

Bordered by volcanoes and geysers, the Puritama Hot Springs sit at the foot of a canyon in the Atacama Desert, 3,475m above sea level. Eight geothermal pools, some of which are fed by waterfalls, are connected via wooden walkways. The high-altitude sodium and sulfate-rich waters are recommended for arthritis, rheumatism and other ailments and stay at a gentle 32 to 33 °C year-round.

DUNTON HOT SPRINGS, COLORADO, USA

Built on the site of an old ghost town, situated in southwestern Colorado, water from the hot springs is wine-red and rich in iron, magnesium and lithium. Used a century ago by miners to soak their weary bones, visitors come to enjoy the wilderness and take a dip in one of six natural baths – all high with mineral content and boasting majestic mountain and meadow views.

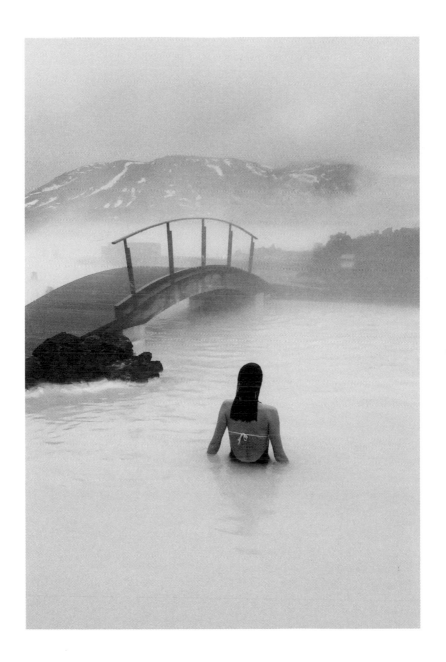

95 Bathe

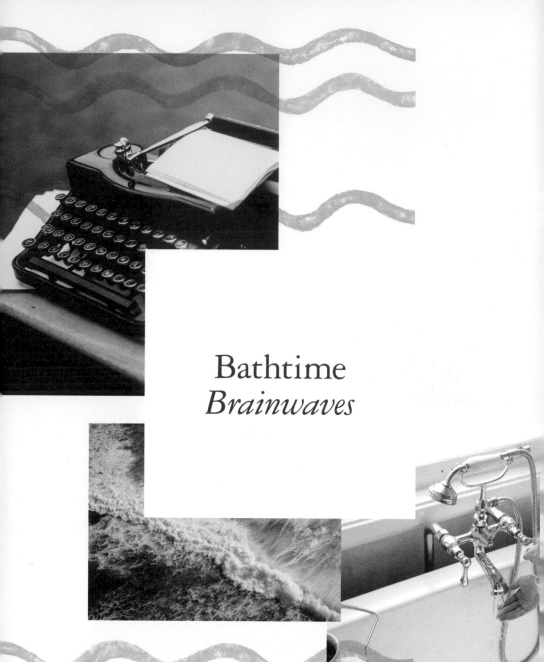

Bathtime
Brainwaves

These notable figures believed that their bath
was a key factor in success and self-care.

[WINSTON CHURCHILL]
1874-1965

The former Prime Minister would take two daily
hot baths to de-stress from the pressures of leading
the country during World War II. Not only were
they important for his well-being but he often
dictated to his secretary, Elizabeth Layton, who
would sit outside the bathroom with a portable
typewriter on her lap. His baths were drawn by his
butler, Mr Inces, and had to be kept at a particular
temperature, measured by a thermometer.

PURIFY

[RICHARD BRANSON]
1950-

This business magnate, philanthropist and co-
founder of The Virgin Group claims his best ideas
are born in the bath and has noted that looking
after ourselves is a key ingredient to success. 'I
like the bath,' he says. 'I love sort of sitting about
relaxing in the bath and having a good think'.

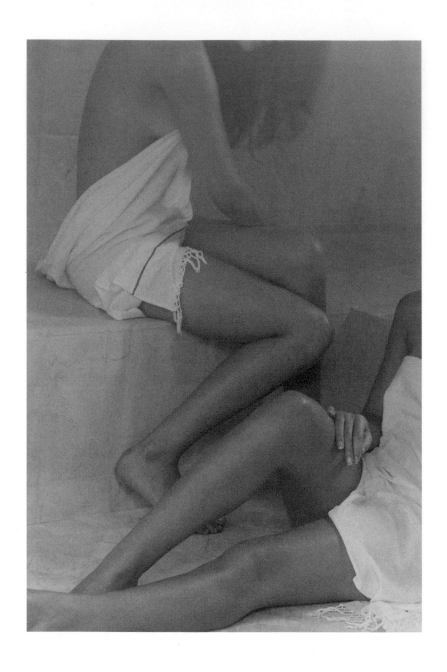

98 Bathe

Some like it hot!
Inside the sauna

According to devotees, a few minutes in a sauna is all that it takes
to look better, feel better and sleep better. Sauna is the only Finnish
word in the English dictionary and it means 'bath' and 'bathhouse'.
Invented in Finland over 2,000 years ago, it is a small wooden room
or house designed as a place to experience dry or wet heat sessions,
bathing the body in dry heat or steam. They are so popular with the
Finns that life without a sauna is unthinkable. In Finland there is one
sauna for every 1.8 people and one per household! Other countries
that love saunas and regularly use them include Sweden, Norway,
Estonia, Germany and Russia.

Traditional saunas were heated by wood, burned by a stove, with
or without a chimney. The latter – known as a 'smoke-sauna' – is the
original Finnish sauna and considered to be the best. The door is
closed when the wood has burned down, leaving the embers to heat
the sauna at the proper temperature. Now, most saunas are heated
by electricity. This source heats the rocks to provide a soft heat and
water is thrown on these rocks to provide humidity. The Finns like their
saunas hot – up to around 100 °C is normal.

After around 10 to 15 minutes of sweating (the average person will
lose around a pint of sweat during a brief sauna session), participants take
a cooling shower, or even a dip in a freezing lake, before repeating the
process. The sauna is not just a place to bathe but is seen as somewhere
to relax, socialise and even do business.

PURIFY

So, what are the benefits of saunas?

- **Reduces stress:** Many sauna users cite stress reduction as the number one reason for using the sauna. The heat, relaxation and technology-free environment stimulate the release of feel-good endorphins.

- **Boosts heart and cardiovascular health:** Being in the sauna gives the heart a workout, and scientific studies have shown that frequent visits are associated with lower death rates from cardiovascular disease and strokes. Earlier studies have also proven that sauna usage benefits people with risk factors for heart disease such as high cholesterol and high blood pressure.

- **Flushes out toxins and clears the skin:** Deep sweating helps to clear the skin of toxins, dead skin cells and impurities, cleansing within the deeper layers. In the polluted world that we live in, a sauna will also aid the kidneys and liver in the process of detoxification. The heat also improves circulation, giving your skin a healthy glow.

- **Soothes aches and relaxes muscles:** Saunas help soothe any aches and pains because of the release of endorphins, which has a mild numbing effect. In one Finnish study, bathing in an infra-red sauna (which uses infra-red light in addition to heat) was shown to help athletes recover from strength and endurance training.

- **Improves immunity:** It has long been proven that sauna use boosts immunity and one recent study has proven that sweating in a sauna at least twice a week could slash the risk of life-threatening infections like pneumonia by almost a third. They are also great for clearing the sinuses and congestion if you suffer from hay fever.

- **Can help with weight loss:** Yes, you can lose weight by sitting and doing nothing! Most people are able to sweat off around 300 to

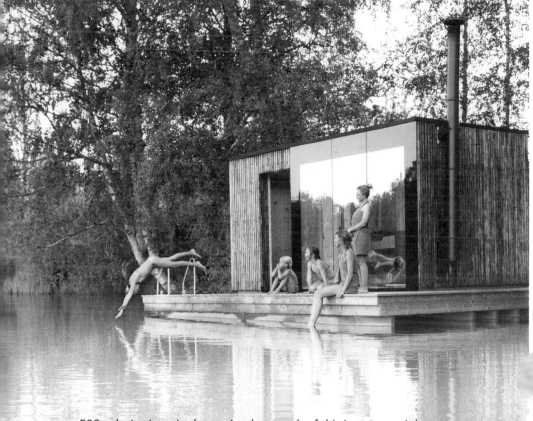

500 calories in a single session but much of this is water weight. By supplementing saunas with cold interludes, this also encourages weight loss. We have two types of fat cells, white and brown, and when we feel cold, brown fat cells work by burning energy to produce heat. By repeating exposure to hot and cold, our brown fat cells are trained to work harder, burning more energy and fat no only when you move from hot to cold environments, but also in normal conditions. This is why hot and cold showering, known as 'contrast therapy', also helps to burn fat.

- **Better sleep:** Research has shown that we can achieve longer and deeper sleep by using saunas because our bodies heat up, then our temperature plummets, inducing a relaxed slumber.

BARE SAUNA FACTS:

FINNISH SAUNA ETIQUETTE

Saunas are considered good for everyone. Only those with serious health conditions should avoid them. They are a place for physical and mental purifying and cleansing – somewhere to kick back and unwind.

Men and women go to saunas separately and families go together but if you are ever unsure, don't be afraid to ask.

Always shower first and wash thoroughly so you keep the sauna clean.

Take off all your clothes – try not to be shy. However, there is no obligation to go nude; wearing a swimsuit or covering up with a towel is acceptable.

Always shut the door behind you so you don't let any cold air in and sit down. The higher benches will be hotter than the lower ones.

Naked skin should not touch the pine benches, so sauna-goers should sit or lie down on a towel. It is more comfortable and hygienic.

Drink lots of water to stay hydrated. In fact, many Finns will eat and drink in saunas; this is considered quite normal.

A bundle of fresh birch twigs – known as *vasta* or *vihta* – might be offered. These are used to gently whip the skin and are said to improve circulation.

A sauna is a place for relaxation, so silence and quiet conversation are both acceptable.

Take a cold plunge:
Ice-bathing after a sauna

The application of heat and ice to muscle injuries has long been used by athletes to aid and speed recovery. In many Nordic cultures, a sauna session is followed by a dip in ice-cold water, a cold shower or even the sea. Some like to roll in the snow and ice swimming is even a popular activity in Finland!

This cold immersion increases the sauna's elevation of heart rate, adrenaline and endorphins and relieves stress and depression. It also improves blood flow, pulling the blood back to your main organs, reinforcing the body's natural defences and helping muscles recover faster.

Many sportspeople swear by ice baths after exercise. They are said to reduce inflammation, constrict blood vessels and flush out waste produce. As the tissue warms, this increases circulation and the healing process is boosted. Bathe in water that is no lower than 15°C, so it won't give you chilblains.

Warm baths are obviously good for sore muscles because the temperature helps muscles relax and stimulates blood supply and metabolism. So what is best? Experiment with ice baths periodically to see how your body responds and what works best for you. If you want to combine bathing and relaxation, a warm bath is probably best!

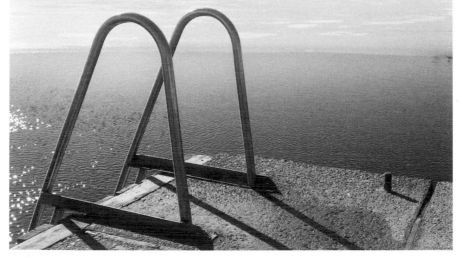

Feeling lonely?
Take a bath

Have you ever referred to someone as being 'warm' or giving you the 'cold shoulder'? Many of us use physical terms when describing people. We take these abstract psychological terms and understand them literally.

Being warm is central to our early lives; babies are cuddled and kissed, held, washed and attended to, and this facilitates bonding and connectedness. Some of the areas in the brain that register physical temperature are also sensitive to emotions around rejection and loneliness.

One study at Yale University in the US showed that having a bath could make you feel less lonely. Researchers asked a group of 400 volunteers, aged 18 to 65, to keep a diary of their bathing habits and note down how they were feeling before and after their bath. Results showed that baths ward off feelings of isolation and indicate that many of us take warm baths to consciously eliminate feelings of being alone. The greater the feelings of loneliness, the longer we stay in the bath and the hotter the temperature. Scientists concluded that the association between warmth and comfort is hardwired in our brains in infancy, explaining why we seek comfort in hot drinks and soup. So, the next time you feel companionless, hop in the tub!

PURIFY

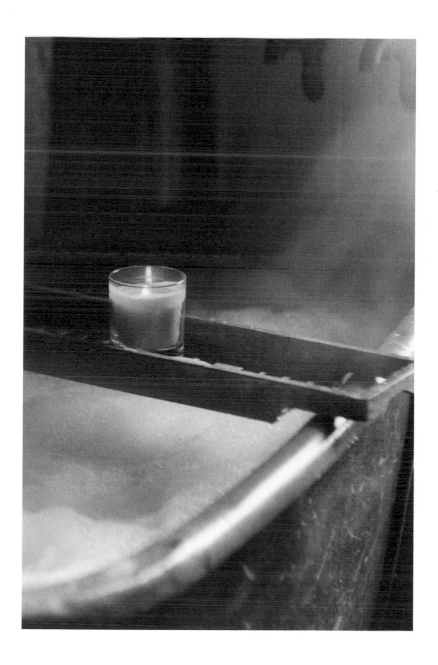

Rejuvenate

'Noble deeds and hot
baths are the best
cures for depression'

[DODIE SMITH, *I CAPTURE THE CASTLE*]

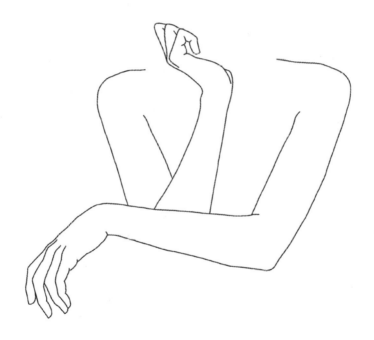

109   Bathe

Bathing is as essential as anything
we do as humans, yet it frequently
gets overlooked in any list of
healing and wellness habits.

While bathing is one of the most important
ways to maintain good health, it is a myth that
we need to bathe regularly; our survival does
not depend on it. However, there are a myriad
of reasons why we bathe. From purifying our skin,
maintaining good health, and protecting ourselves
from infections and illnesses through to improving
our self-confidence and physical well-being and
easing emotional stress, the bath is an important
tool for rejuvenation and wellness.

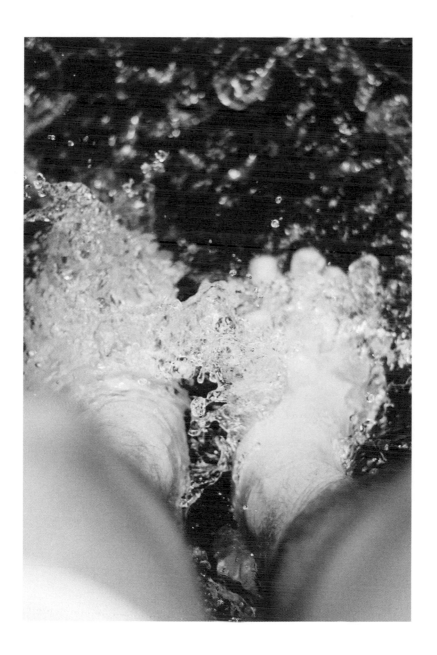

111   Bathe

Bathing:
The Science

Since ancient times, bathing in water has been equated with physical and mental health, and the science speaks for itself. There is even a term for the practice – balneotherapy – which means the treatment of disease through bathing.

- **Improves circulation and heart health:** Taking a hot bath will make your heart work faster and become stronger, giving it a healthy workout and improving circulation. This increases sweating so will help to eliminate toxins, viruses and bacteria from the body.

- **Relieves muscle aches and pains:** Baths have always been a tonic for aching muscles. This is because they raise the temperature of sore muscles and block pain receptors, producing pain relief. For athletes, who have cold baths after exercise, this lowers the levels of lactic acid in the bloodstream, so muscles can recover faster.

- **Calms the nervous system:** Bathing reduces stress and anxiety and can boost mood. A study at the University of Wolverhampton found that a daily bath, usually at the end of the day, significantly improved the mood and optimism of the participants.

- **Burns calories:** Excess fat is associated with multiple health problems, including heart disease, diabetes and more. Experts at Loughborough University found that sitting for an hour in a hot bath lowered blood sugar levels more effectively than spending the same amount of time cycling, benefiting people with type 2 diabetes.

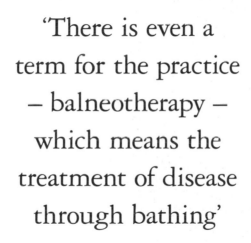

'There is even a
term for the practice
– balneotherapy –
which means the
treatment of disease
through bathing'

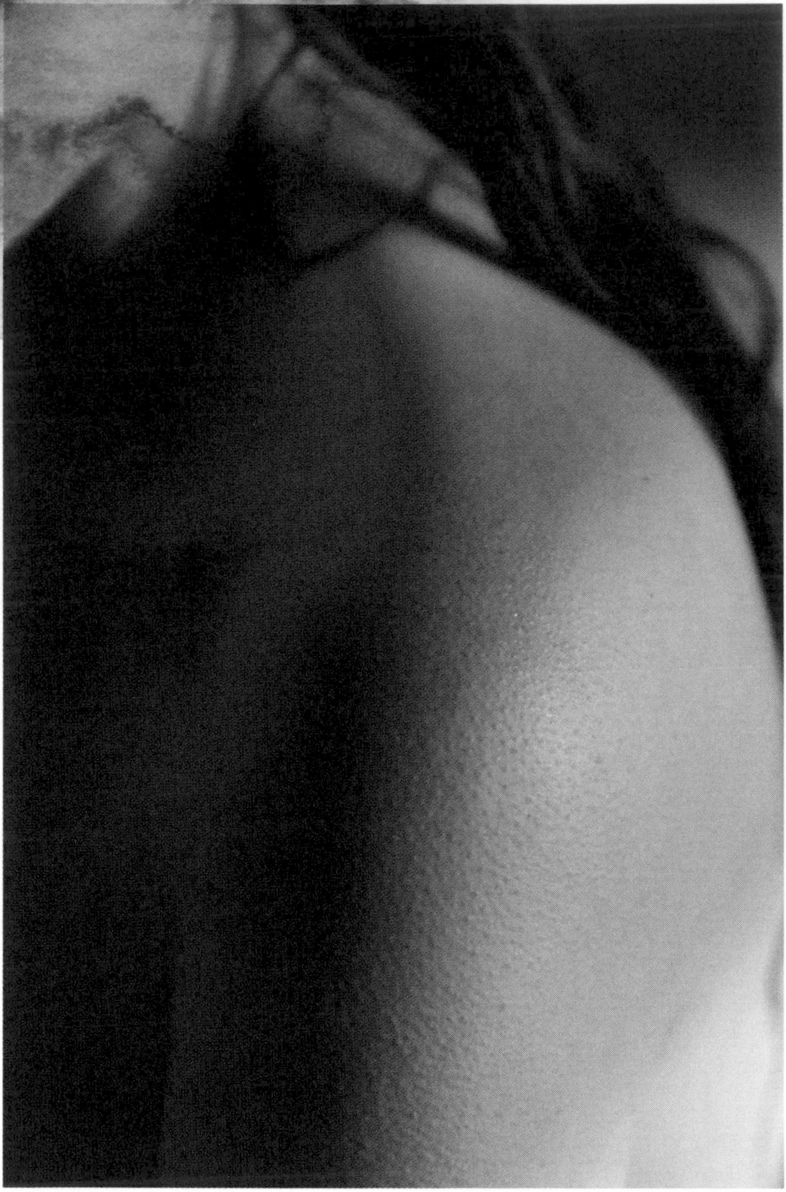

REJUVENATE

- **Lowers blood pressure:** Studies have proven that bathing significantly lowers blood pressure. For those with high blood pressure, this is particularly important and will lower their risk of having a stroke, improve vision and boost kidney health.

- **Helps with coughs and colds:** The best way to reduce inflammation and dry out mucus in the nasal passages and throat is to help clear them with steam. A 2011 study also found that elevated body temperature can help certain elements of the immune system to function more efficiently, warding off infections and viruses.

- **Aids sleep:** A good night's sleep is associated with everything from weight control to better immunity and pain recovery, and baths are long proven to help the body drift off.

- **Benefits muscles, joints and bones:** Moving in water has been shown to lessen impact on joints, muscles and bones; it also improves postural stability.

REJUVENATE

What is a Turkish hammam?

A Turkish bath or hammam is a public bath; it is closely related to ancient Roman and Greek baths and is a place of renowned rejuvenation of the physical, mental and even spiritual kind. It is believed that the Ottoman Turks inherited the bathing concept and adapted it to Turkish tastes. The word 'hammam' originates from the Arabic 'hamma', which means 'heating up'. Sometimes hammams are referred to as Turkish baths, and are a major part of their culture, used for cleansing and relaxing. Traditionally, they can be found all over Turkey and in Arabic, North African and Eastern countries. Often they are located near a mosque because Muslims wash themselves before prayer.

Males and females are separated in traditional hammams because Islam preaches modesty in relations between men and women, but the hammam experience is the same for both sexes. Because of this, nudity is common, though bathing suits are also worn.

Some hammams have one tiled room, while others have a suite of rooms of differing temperatures. On arrival, guests are given a woven cloth used to cover the body. The experience begins with relaxation before entering a heated, tiled room with a warm marble platform in the centre, situated under a domed ceiling. Small sinks around the side have hot and cold running water so the temperature can be adjusted but they tend to be very hot and humid; unlike saunas, there is a lot of moisture and steam. Visitors spread their towels on the hot central navel stone and lie down on their stomachs to allow the heat to penetrate their pores and help their muscles to relax.

Now, visitors are ready for the massage! They are exfoliated by an attendant with a handwoven wash cloth – known as a 'kese' – and scrubbed, which boosts circulation and sloughs away dead skin. Then comes the foam massage, where guests are vigorously massaged using foam before being washed or showered down with cold water. In traditional hammams, they also offer a balloon soap massage, where foam is squeezed over the body from an air- and soap-filled pillowcase. The sensation is soft and fluffy, like being cleaned by a cloud!

In most hammams, the washing spaces are separated by marble panels, making the experience a more private one. Some hammams offer slightly differing treatments but all aim for a ritual accessing well-being. Most hammams then offer Turkish tea, so guests can stay hydrated and enjoy the feeling of calm and vitality.

The Rhassoul ritual

Rhassoul, sometimes called rasul or ghassoul, comes from the word 'ghassala', which means 'to wash'. This is a traditional Arabic body treatment, which is often applied by Moroccan women after the hammam. This healing clay, sourced from the Atlas Mountains of Morocco, is enriched with plant and herb extracts. For years, many women used rhassoul for soap, shampoo and skin conditioner. It is applied to the hair and skin after cleansing the warm room and rinsed away after around ten to 15 minutes. This removes toxins and impurities from the skin and nourishes it too.

REJUVENATE

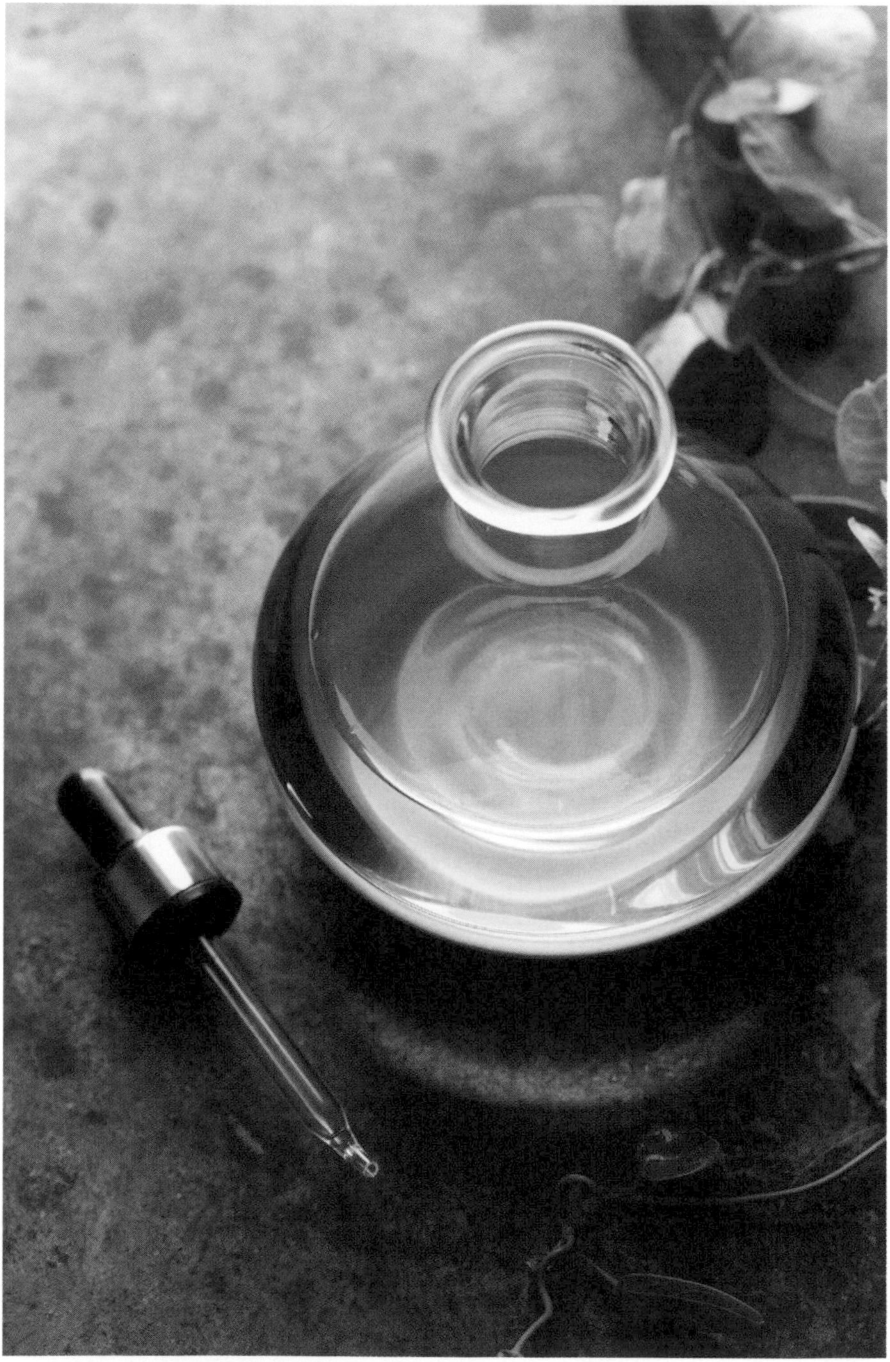

HOW TO GET THE HAMMAM GLOW AT HOME

The beneficial components of the hammam ritual include the warm and steamy air, the vigorous exfoliation and a therapeutic massage – a combination which works to deeply cleanse and purify the body and will leave your skin as smooth as silk.

Create steam: Create your own sauna-like atmosphere by letting the hot shower run until the room becomes steamy and warm. If you wish, add a few drops of essential oils to a diffuser to create an aromatic scent. Pregnant women are advised to not use steam rooms or certain oils.

Soap it up: Moroccan black soap, which has a paste-like structure, is used in many hammams and has both anti-bacterial and invigorating properties. Lather up all over.

Exfoliate: A central part of the hammam ritual. Authentic hammam-style gloves are available to buy or use a normal scrubbing mitt to slough away dead skin cells. Massage in circular motions before rinsing.

Purify: If you wish (this is an optional step), massage a thin layer of deep-cleansing body mud into the skin to polish it intensively, leaving it clean and fresh. Keep it on for a few minutes before washing off.

Moisturise: After rinsing, apply moisturising body oil directly onto the skin. There are many suitable body oils on the market; a good option is nourishing argan oil, which is rich in vitamins A and E.

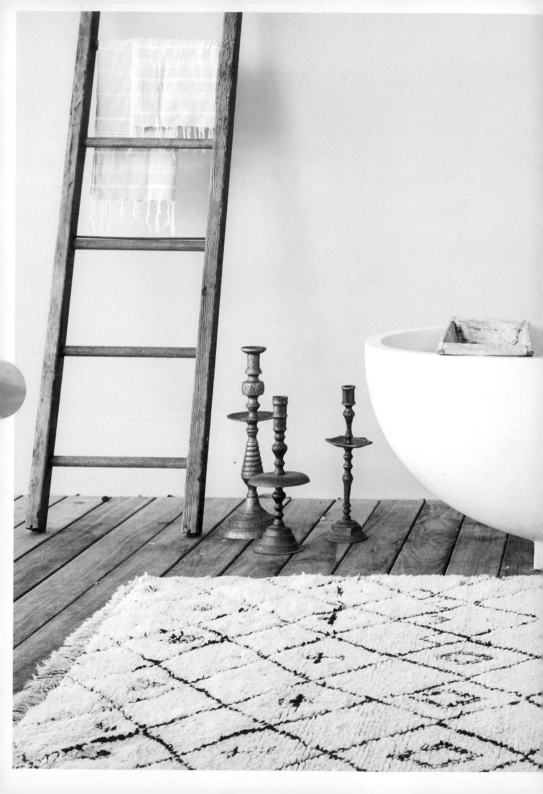

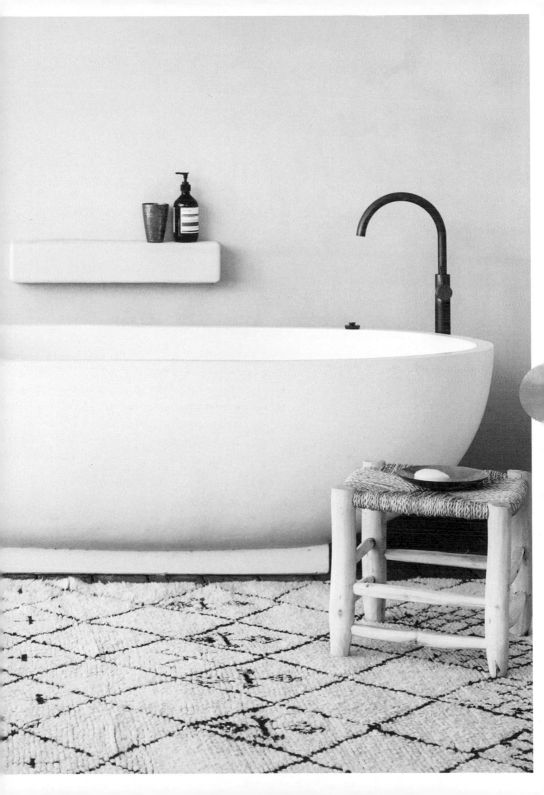

Is taking a hot bath
as good as exercise?

Go for a run or run a bath? We all know that exercise and sweating is good for us, but can you reap the benefits without hitting the treadmill? Can passive heating, as opposed to sweating through exercise, benefit us?

One recent study at Loughborough University looked at the effects of taking hot baths versus exercise. Researchers measured blood sugar control, an indicator of metabolic fitness, and calories burnt during one hour of cycling compared to an hour-long bath at 40°C. These activities were designed to raise the core body temperature by 1°C over the hour. The 14 male participants taking part in the study had their blood sugar measured for 24 hours afterwards.

Cycling burned more calories than bathing but the bathers burnt around 140 calories, the same as a half-hour walk. The blood sugar results for both parties were almost identical but peak blood sugar after eating was about 10 per cent lower when the men took a hot bath, compared to exercise. Researchers also showed that the anti-inflammatory response after having a bath is similar to after exercise. This helps us fight off infection and disease and can reduce chronic inflammation associated with illnesses such as type 2 diabetes.

It is acknowledged that wider research is needed in the field of 'passive heating' but this study has shown how a family of proteins referred to as 'health shock proteins' are produced in the body in response to physically stressful circumstances, such as exercise and passive heating. These proteins are thought to assist with the function of insulin and improve blood sugar control. This research backs up previous studies showing that frequent sauna use reduces the risk of strokes and heart attacks, and that regular baths can improve blood pressure. Perhaps this is not a reason to stop exercising, but definitely another reason to hop in the bath!

'This research backs up previous studies showing that frequent sauna use reduces the risk of strokes and heart attacks, and that regular baths can improve blood pressure'

Thalassotherapy
for healing

Thalassotherapy comes from the Greek words 'thalosso' meaning sea and 'therapia' meaning treatment. The concept, invented by Frenchman Jacques de la Bonnardière during the 1860s, channels the healing and beneficial properties of the sea. Throughout Europe, seawater and thalassotherapy have been used for centuries as treatments for muscle and joint complaints.

There are a number of thalassotherapy centres around the world that focus on using mineral-rich seawater and marine-based products, which are rich in antioxidants and trace elements. Treatments may include: Spa baths, where thousands of bubbles provide a re-mineralising massage; seaweed baths; affusion showers (a shower with a rain-like spray, which is designed to massage the body); hydro-massages; jet massages; seaweed wraps; and cryotherapy, where the lower limbs are wrapped in seaweed to boost circulation.

'Seawater and
thalassotherapy
have been used
for centuries as
treatments
for muscle and
joint complaints'

REJUVENATE

BATHTIME YOGA:

FIVE BATHTIME STRETCHES

Add some yoga to your bathtime routine to deepen the effects of a dip. Follow these simple stretches, allowing the warmth of the water to help you unwind.

NECK ROLLS

This soothing and dynamic warm-up technique will stretch the neck muscles and cervical spine (the part of the neck housing the spinal cord) and can help alleviate stiffness associated with neck strain. This is especially good if you have been sitting at a desk for long periods.

Sit in the bath with your hands and arms on your knees.
As you inhale, gently tilt your head to the right and start rolling it back.
Keep rolling your head to the left and then down.
Bring your head back to a neutral position and repeat in the
    opposite direction.

SHOULDER ROLLS

This movement will relieve tension in the upper back and shoulders, and improve circulation in these joints.

Sit upright in the bath and as you inhale, lift your shoulders to your ears.
As you exhale, slowly roll your shoulders round and back, dropping them
    away from your ears.
If you wish, you can do each shoulder alternately before practising with
    both shoulders together.

SEATED CAT COW (UPAVISTHA BITILASANA MARJARYASANA)

This pose stretches the muscles at the hip, back and abdomen, expands the lungs and chest and aligns the spine.

Sit upright in the bath and roll your shoulder blades back and down with your arms relaxed on your knees.

As you inhale, arch your back, leading with your chest, and look towards the ceiling (the Cow pose). Lift your chin and keep your arms relaxed.

As you exhale, round your spine and let your head drop forwards (the Cat pose). Tuck in your chin and allow your shoulders to roll forwards.

Repeat five more times, moving seamlessly from Cat to Cow with each breath.

SIMPLE SEATED TWIST (PARIVRTTA SUKHASANA)

If you're not accustomed to twisting your body, this easy pose is the perfect way to start. Stretching the upper chest, shoulders and back, this twist also tones the organs in the abdomen, improves metabolism and energises the nervous system.

Sit upright, midway down the bath, with your legs crossed (as much as your flexibility and bathtub allows). Be sure to sit up tall and elongate your spine.

As you inhale, place your right hand flat against the floor of the bath behind you and your left hand on your right knee.

As you exhale, try to move deeper into the twist and look over your right shoulder.

Hold for five breaths and repeat on the other side.

SEATED FORWARD BEND (PASCHIMOTTANASANA)

This seated forward bend will completely stretch the back muscles and hamstrings. It also stimulates the reproductive and urinary systems and calms the nervous system.

Sit in the bath with your legs straight out in front of you.

Press down through your heels and as you inhale, lift your arms above your head.

Hinging at the hips, lower your torso towards the legs, leading with the chest.

Reach for your toes, feet or ankles.

To deepen the stretch, gently pull your toes towards you or use your arms to pull your torso closer to your legs.

Breathe and hold for five breaths.

As you release the pose, slowly roll up the spine back into a sitting position.

Bathing through the seasons

Bathing should not be confined to the cold winter months. Emotional and physical immersions can help connect mind, body and soul to the seasons. Tune in by taking note of what is going on in nature and mirror this with your bathtime. This will help you to harness the power of each season in more ways than you can imagine… not just by changing what you put into the bath, but also the time of day, the duration and temperature of your bath.

WINTER

Winter weather is synonymous with the need for a warming, reviving hot bath. Frosty mornings, icy evenings and arriving home, having been caught in a rain shower, all cry out for baths that warm, revive and soothe.

Banish draughts from the room, close curtains or blinds and spark up your private piece of sunshine by lighting candles. For a liquid winter warmer, try to draw the bath 20 minutes before you want to get in, adding pure essential oils to suit the weather and the mood; their scent will wind its way through the house. Close the door to create a cocoon of comfort and intensify the olfactory effects of the oils, at the same time turning your bathroom into an Eastern hammam or Turkish bath, full of steam and sensual aromas.

But which oils to use? Traditionally, winter calls for warming choices, but you can also conjure up the spruce-scented bliss of a crisp alpine day with a simple combination of pine, eucalyptus and juniper oils. Medicinal roots dug up in autumn sustain us at this time: ginger, echinacea and horseradish keep our blood warm and our immune systems strong, so why not mimic this kitchen wisdom in the bathroom?

Other warming oils include black pepper, cardamom, cedarwood, cypress, fir needle, juniper berry, peppermint, pine needle, wintergreen and rosemary. Try making up your own blends using a muslin pouch and filling it with freshly bruised herbs or add a few drops of oil to the bath after it has filled (adding oils to a running bath will cause them to evaporate so add after your bath is drawn to harness their power). These oils are also a great way to improve circulation, ease muscular pain and warm up cold hands and feet, as well as helping to minimise the symptoms of colds and coughs.

If you want a blend that's less pine-and-herb-laden, other great winter oils are cinnamon, clove, orange, lemon and black spruce. Bergamot is a great oil if you're feeling the winter blues, as is clary sage. And, in the run-up to Christmas, soothe your festive stresses with a few drops of royally good frankincense, which is so powerful it can help relieve chronic stress and anxiety, reduce pain and inflammation, and boost immunity – the ultimate winter tonic.

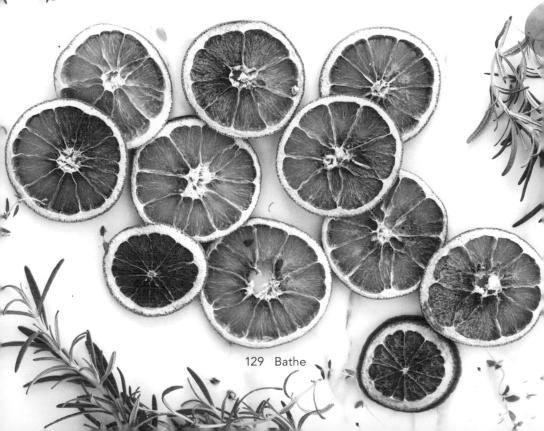

SPRING

As the evenings start to become lighter, we feel a sense of new growth, renewed, increased energy and a fresh sense of purpose. At this time of year, don't forgo your bathing ritual for the rush of the shower though. Instead, see your bath as a chance to stimulate, energise and enliven. Spring is when our hot, bright, active yang energies come to the fore (the ancient Chinese philosophy of how 'dark-bright' and 'negative-positive': contrary forces may actually be complementary, interconnected and interdependent in the natural world, and how they may give rise to each other as they interrelate to one another). Yang denotes light, warmth and activity amongst other things and is beginning to rise at this time. Shake off the sleepiness of winter and embrace the renewed vitality of spring – a spring bath can accelerate this.

However, bathtime in spring may mean a cooler water temperature and a quicker, more cleansing experience, compared with the hibernating long, slow immersions of winter. Oils for spring reflect the fact that flowers are starting to bud. It's time to think fresh and green so bring in natural and organic body scrubs and pre-bath dry body brushing to remove the remnants of winter from the skin (again, always go for natural products so that you are not soaking in a toxic soup!).

If possible, bring the outside in by opening curtains and blinds to maximise light or even opening a window to let in a little fresh spring air – if you can hear birdsong, so much the better as it is another proven, natural relaxant. Place vases of fresh spring flowers or pots of scented bulbs around the bathroom for a splash of seasonal colour.

A great oil blend for spring is four drops of sweet orange, four drops of petitgrain and eight drops of neroli sprinkled into a drawn bath. In the garden it's a time when flowers and leaves appear and the life force is at its most potent. Match this liveliness with fresh, green, uplifting oils in the bath, such as peppermint, bergamot, citronella, lavender, jasmine, ylang ylang and basil.

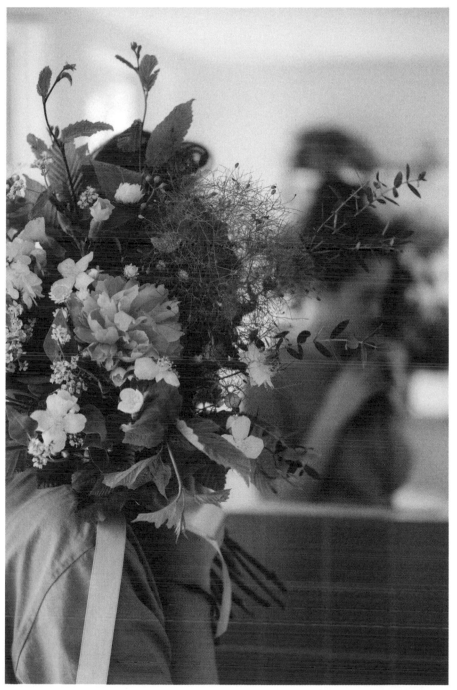

SUMMER

Continued growth typifies the summer months – a time for being outside as much as possible, socialising and looking outwards rather than inwards. In nature, green is the colour, as herbs run riot, flowers fill gardens with scent and colour, and the sun is at its highest and brightest. Our energy levels, too, are at their height, so an uplifting bath is most beneficial if it can compliment these, rather than slowing us down, as in winter. Alternatively, and here is where tuning into your own energy levels is key, if your energy is off the radar, bring it down to more manageable levels with your choice of bath oils – your sense of smell will be the best diagnosis as to what you need. Go with your nose!

Summer is also a time of hedonistic pleasure, vibrancy and light, so reflect this in your bath. Warmer months are the perfect time to diffuse and blend your own bouquet, with light, energising, herbaceous, floral and cooling essential oils like the variety of a summer garden: mint, citrus and floral elements with geranium, jasmine, basil, neroli, citrus, lemon balm, peppermint and camomile. During the summer it may seem more tempting to take a shower rather than have a bath, but a bath is still a joy: use cooler water, open the windows wide and luxuriate in a feeling of light, air and refreshing cleansing.

'Your sense of smell will be the best diagnosis as to what you need. Go with your nose!'

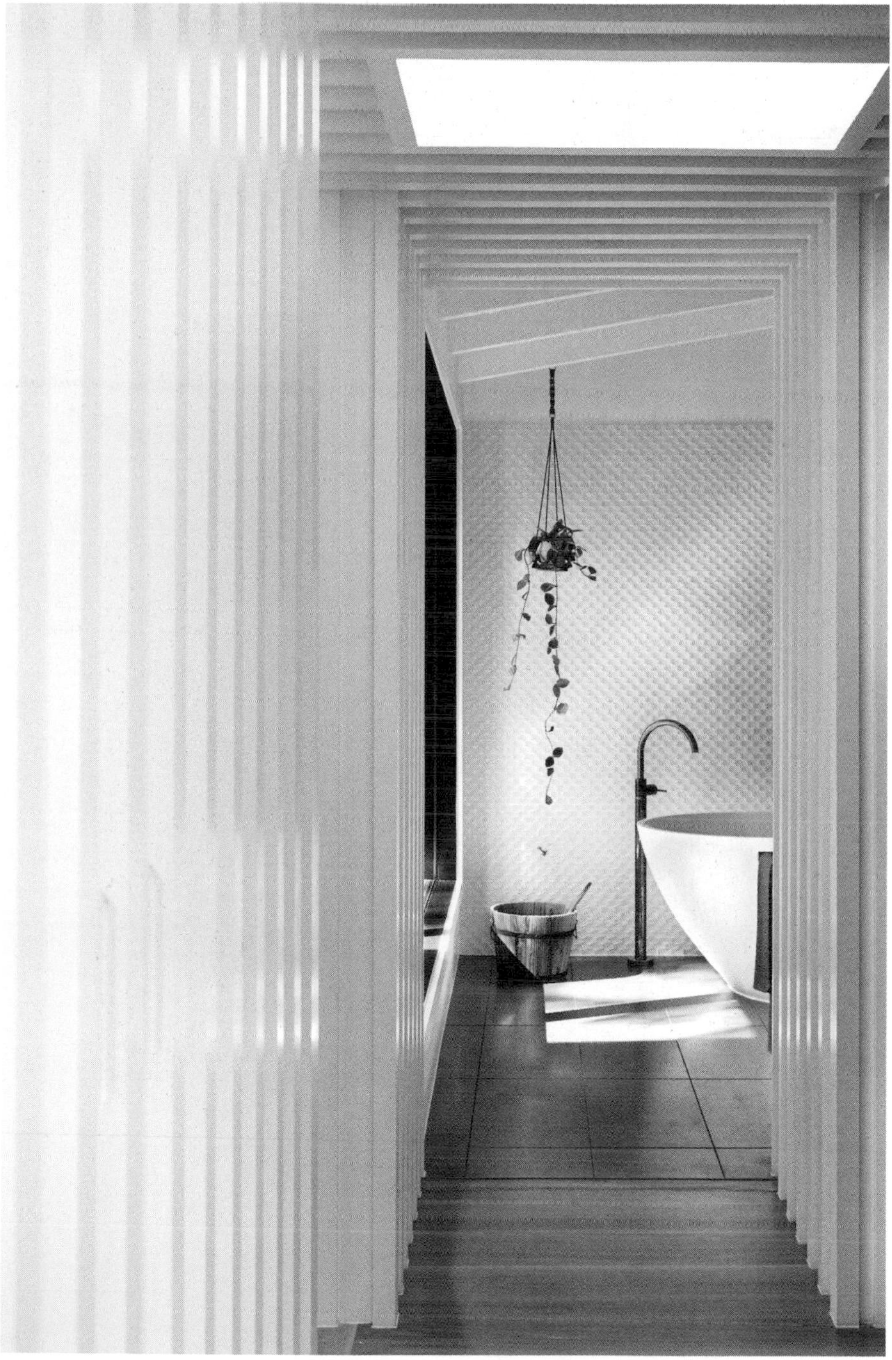

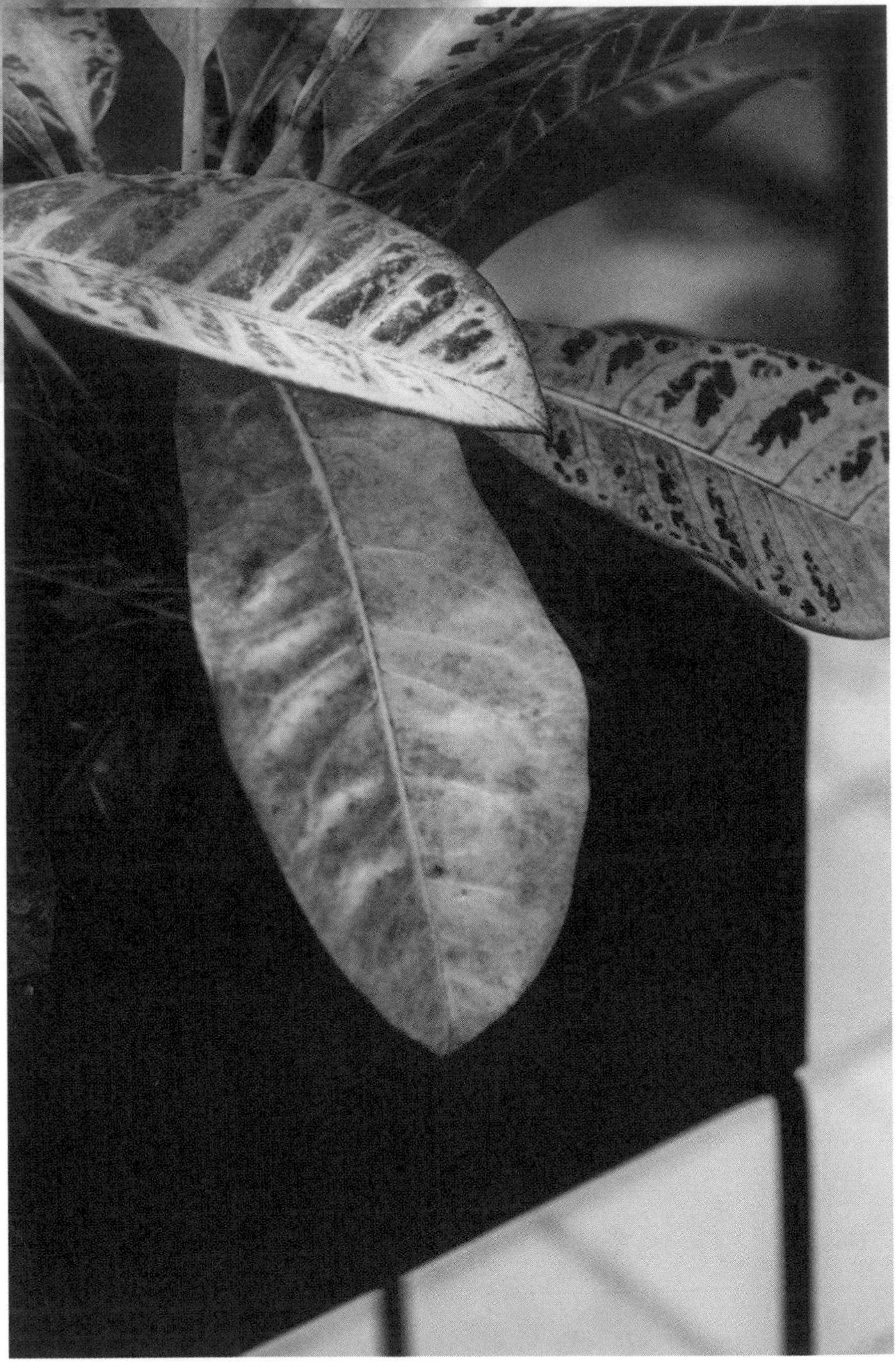

AUTUMN

Following the heady heat of the summer, take a lead from nature and slow down. Autumn heralds a time to take stock and appreciate the abundance of the summer harvest, the earth's bounty, the ebb and flow of nature, our community and all that we are grateful for, as we prepare for the leaner times of winter. Not surprisingly, a relaxing bath is one of the best ways to ease into autumn, turning our attention to the home as the days shorten. And, as the temperature lowers, what better opportunity to lower yourself into a wonderful autumn bath, increasing the heat of the water as the air cools outside? As autumn makes way for winter, you can turn up the hot tap.

When thinking about the oils to use, (in the bath, or in diffusers and burners) again think about the seasonal foods we like to eat at this time of year – spices such as cinnamon, ginger, nutmeg and cloves and citrus fruits such as oranges are starting to make an appearance and these work just as well in the bath, as does juniper, fir, pine and rosemary. A wonderful autumn blend is four drops of bergamot oil, eight drops of geranium oil and two drops of rose oil. Inspired by the hedgerows, you could also try rosehip seed oil and place a vase of colourful autumn leaves in the bathroom or a vibrant-coloured autumnal pot plant.

Other oils that suit the scents and emotions of autumn are cinnamon and patchouli, as well as energising citrus oils: bergamot, sweet orange, mandarin and tangerine, with lime, lemon and grapefruit.

Many people feel sadness at the ending of the summer – if so, clary sage, sandalwood, frankincense and bergamot are all good at helping us to accept change and allaying anxiety and depression, as are sweet orange and lemon oils, which keep the summer feeling and uplift the mind and soul.

REJUVENATE

Baths with a difference: Weird baths from around the world

Baths are good for the soul. But not all baths are filled with water. If you fancy a soak in beer or green tea, there are places you can go to take an unusual dip.

BEER BATHS

In lager-loving hotspots, the beer is considered so good that visitors are invited to bathe in it! Select breweries and spas in Austria, the Czech Republic, Germany, Colorado and Iceland are taking advantage of beer's skin-friendly vitamins, proteins and carbohydrates. Guests soak in beer, water, hops and yeast for around 20 minutes, which is said to be cleansing for the skin and has a positive impact on health.

CHOCOLATE BATHS

At Hotel Hershey in Pennsylvania, managed by the chocolate manufacturer, there is a range of chocolate-based spa treatments to enjoy. The treatments list includes a chocolate fondue wrap, a chocolate sugar scrub, a cocoa massage or the whipped cocoa bath, where guests spend 15 minutes relaxing in a bath of foaming chocolate milk. Chocolate is reputed to be packed with antioxidants, vitamins and minerals.

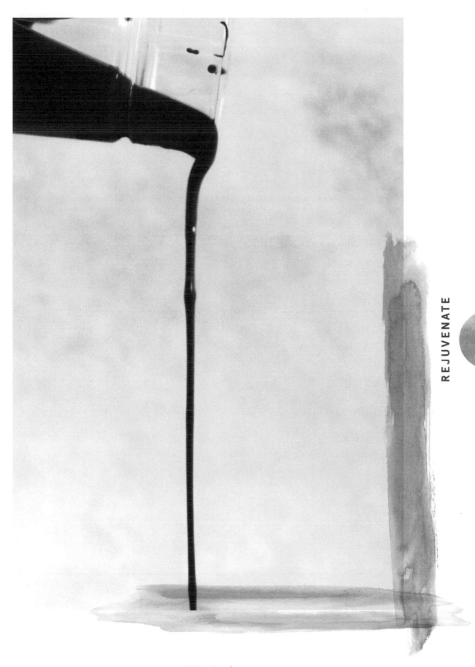

REJUVENATE

137 Bathe

VOLCANO MUD BATH

Unlike a volcano filled with lava, a crater of a dormant volcano in Totumo, Colombia, is filled with natural, dense mud. According to local legend, a priest sprinkled the active volcano, which was spewing molten lava, with holy water, and turned it into mud. There is room for around ten to 15 people and the thick mud is said to be rejuvenating and healing. After bathing, a local attendant will give you a massage and wash you down.

GREEN TEA, COFFEE, SAKE, RED WINE AND RAMEN NOODLE BATHS

After centuries of traditional onsen bathing, Yunessun Spa Resort in Hakone, located 100km west of Tokyo, has branched out into more exotic bathing options, such as green tea, red wine, sake and coffee baths. There is even a pepper-water filled ramen noodle bath. The coffee is brewed in pots and poured in, one barrel at a time, five times a day, while the wine bath includes a 12-foot bottle of wine, so visitors can sip as they bathe. According to Yunessun, these baths go beyond the novelty factor; soaking in sake is good for the skin, green tea boosts the immune system and has antioxidant properties, while coffee provides an energy boost.

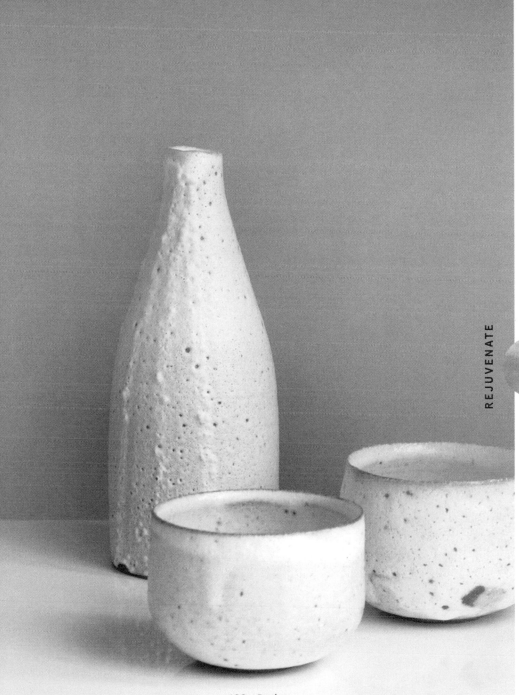

139   Bathe

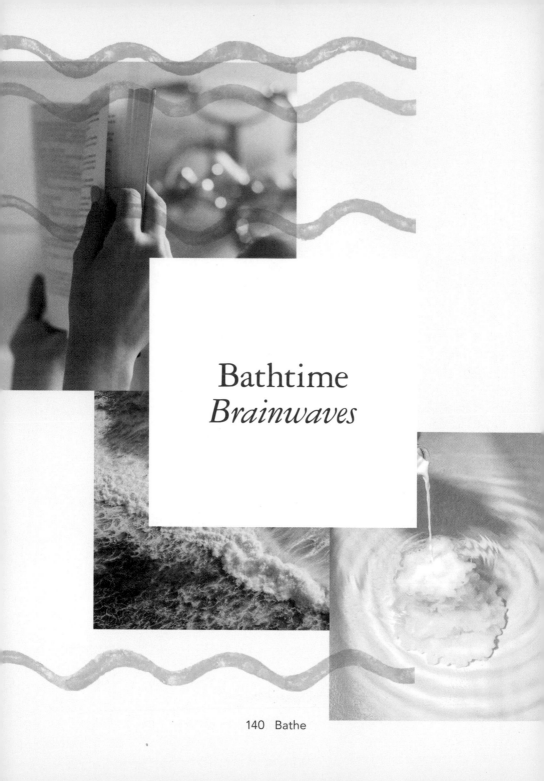

Bathtime
Brainwaves

More famous creative thinkers throughout history.
These familiar faces also found solace, stress relief
and motivation while taking a dip.

[VIRGINIA WOOLF]
1882-1941

The novelist conceived many of her greatest ideas
in the bathtub, including the idea for her novel,
The Years. She said as she soaked, she dreamt up
'an entirely new book – a sequel to *A Room of
One's Own* about the sexual life of women…'

[OPRAH WINFREY]
1954-

The talk show host, actress, producer and
philanthropist is a huge fan of bathing and says:
'I major in bathtubs. I spend my time looking
for the best bathtub a woman can buy.' She also
adores creating bathing experiences, adding
milks, salts and bath gels.

REJUVENATE

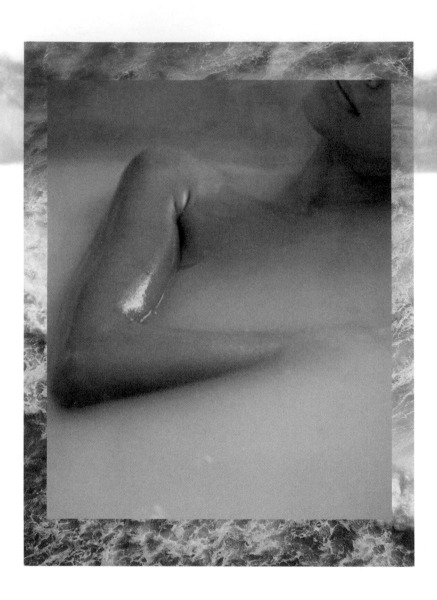

Why do we go wrinkly in the bath?

Do you know why the skin on human fingers and toes shrivels up like a prune when we soak in the bath? For a long time, it was believed that the water passed through the outer layer of the skin, causing it to swell up and become puffy. However, scientists now believe that this could be the result of an autonomic nervous system reaction; this is the system that controls breathing, heart rate and perspiration. The distinctive wrinkling is caused by blood vessels restricting below the skin's surface and it is believed to have an evolutionary function; it is easier to pick objects up or climb out of wet places with wrinkly hands and fingers because they give you more grip.

'It is easier to pick objects up with wrinkly fingers because they give you more grip'

[THREE]

Ritual

'There must be quite
a few things a hot bath
won't cure, but I don't
know many of them...

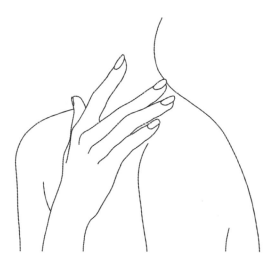

147   Bathe

...Whenever I'm sad, I'm going to die, or so nervous I can't sleep, or in love with somebody I won't be seeing for a week, I slump down just so far and then I say: 'I'll go take a hot bath' I meditate in the bath. The water needs to be very hot, so hot you can barely stand putting your foot in it. Then you lower yourself, inch by inch, until the water's up to your neck.

I remember the ceiling over every bathtub I've stretched out in. I remember the texture of the ceilings, the cracks, the colours, the damp spots and the light fixtures. I remember the tubs, too: The antique griffin-legged tubs, and the modern coffin-shaped tubs, and the fancy pink marble tubs overlooking indoor lily ponds, and I remember the shapes and sizes of the water taps and the different sorts of soap holders. I never feel so much myself as when I'm in a hot bath.'

[FROM SYLVIA PLATH'S *THE BELL JAR*]

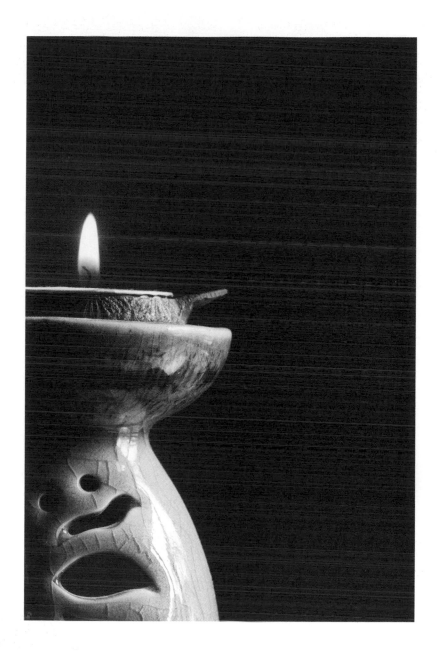

149 Bathe

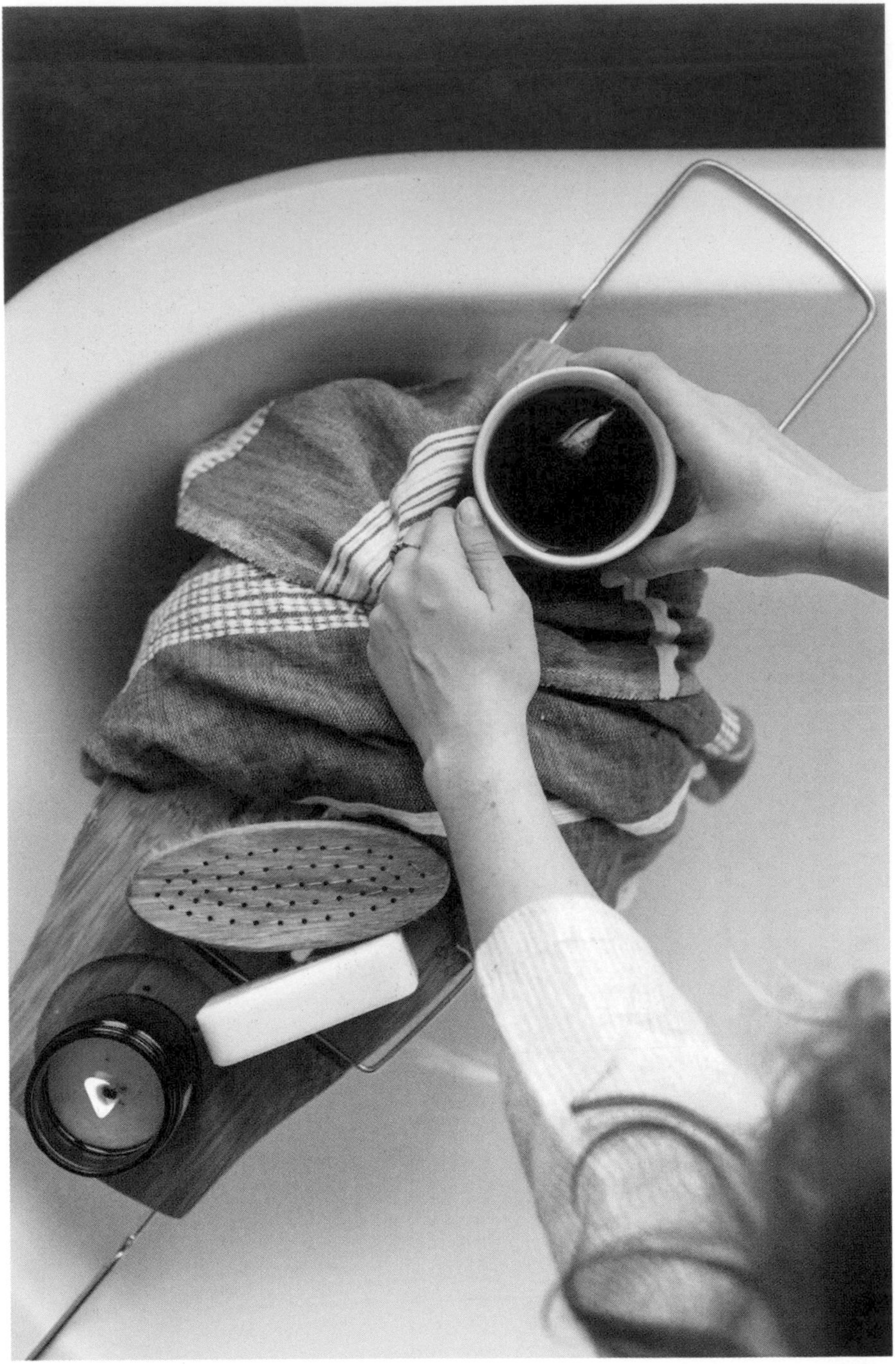

Reframe your bathtime: How to create your own personal bathing ritual

The act of bathing and washing is a personal one, so take your bathing to the next level, giving it a ritualistic quality that is unique to you.

- **Pick your 'magic' time:** The most important part of your ritual is regularity, carving out the time once or twice a week. Allow yourself around 15 to 20 minutes to bathe and time to relax afterwards. Permit yourself the time and schedule it in your diary, like you would an important meeting. You may choose to bathe in the morning before your family are awake, or in the evening to unwind from the stresses of the day. Invest in a 'Do Not Disturb' sign so that flatmates, other halves and children stay out and refrain from asking you questions through the door or playing loud music.

- **Get the temperature right:** Aim for your water to be 36 to 38°C and the room temperature also plays an important role (25 to 30°C is about right). If necessary, heat the room up beforehand because you don't want to put your body under unnecessary stress if there is an excessive temperature difference when you get out.

- **Don't overdo it:** Bathe for 15 to 20 minutes. Staying in the bath too long can dry out your skin and put a strain on the circulatory system. If you are a fan of cold baths, don't stay in for long – take a quick dip before heating yourself up.

- **Supercharge your water:** Whether you enjoy Epsom Salt baths, essential oils, or other natural ingredients, separate or combined, experiment until you find the perfect bath blend for you.

- **Set the mood:** Low lights tell your mind and body to calm down. Either use low lights or turn them off and light some candles. Always opt for natural waxes to keep the air pure. Did you know that when burned, paraffin wax (made from petroleum waste) creates toxic benzene and toluene chemicals, both of which are known carcinogens? If you suffer from headaches when a candle is burning, it may well be down to the paraffin. Plus, the artificial scents and dyes often used can also release harmful chemicals when burned, possibly triggering allergies.

- **Play music if you wish but go tech-free:** Relaxing, classical music can make the perfect bathing companion. Leave all other electronics outside the bathroom door.

- **Quieten your mind:** Whether you practise meditation, or simply want to let your thoughts float away, be aware of keeping your mind calm and still. That 'Do Not Disturb' sign doubles as a powerful, symbolic mental sign-off to you, too.

- **Pamper yourself:** Whether you want to cleanse your body from head to toe, apply a face mask, or deep condition your hair, use some time to practise self-care and indulge your body.

- **Take a moment:** Always finish your bathing ritual slowly and with great care. Use the fluffiest towel you can find to pat yourself dry and take a moment to relax. Afterwards, continue to put any worries aside, mute your phone and read a book, lie down or meditate to allow body and mind to absorb the bathing bliss.

SEVEN EASY WAYS TO SPRUCE

UP YOUR BATHROOM

Whether there are children coming or going, your partner leaves their towels strewn all over the place, or you haven't managed to update the space for a few years, the chances are your bathroom might need a facelift. The bathroom should be one of the most private spaces in any home but how it looks really affects its functionality and how it makes us feel. Here are some simple ideas to turn it into a luxurious sanctuary without a complete refit.

DE-CLUTTER

From almost-empty conditioner bottles through to tatty sponges and rusty razors, if your bathing space is a mess, it's time for a blitz! If anything hasn't been used for six months, check expiry dates and where necessary, throw it away. Keep surfaces as clear as possible.

REFRESH YOUR TOWELS

When was the last time you bought new towels? They are a great investment because you use them every day and you can colour-code them for ease.

CREATIVE STORAGE

Many bathrooms are small, so if you do not have cupboards to hide your toiletries and other products away, use storage creatively. Add pull-out shelves to deep cupboards to keep necessities ordered and easily accessible, and hang baskets on the wall for hand towels, washcloths and other bathing essentials.

UPDATE THE HARDWARE

Rusty handles on drawers and dirty knobs on cabinets can be replaced quickly and easily, giving your bathroom a facelift in the process. Clear, glossy hardware will create a streamlined, minimalist look, while heavier metal pieces will give your bathroom a more rustic feel.

HANG ARTWORK OR A NEW MIRROR

The bathroom should be treated like any other room in your house. Give it an instant boost by hanging some carefully chosen framed (bathroom-friendly) artwork or a new, oversized mirror to make the room look bigger than it is. Let these pieces become a focal point to add to and accessorise around.

REPLACE OUTDATED LIGHTING

Outdated or unflattering bathroom lighting can be easily updated for a warmer or softer lightbulb or even a new statement lighting fixture. Avoid cold, fluorescent lighting and bulbs that are too yellow.

PAINT

A lick of paint on the walls is one of the easiest and most inexpensive ways to really change the look of a room. Make sure you choose a non-toxic paint and a formula designed for moist conditions, and select a colour for its mood-altering as well as aesthetic appeal.

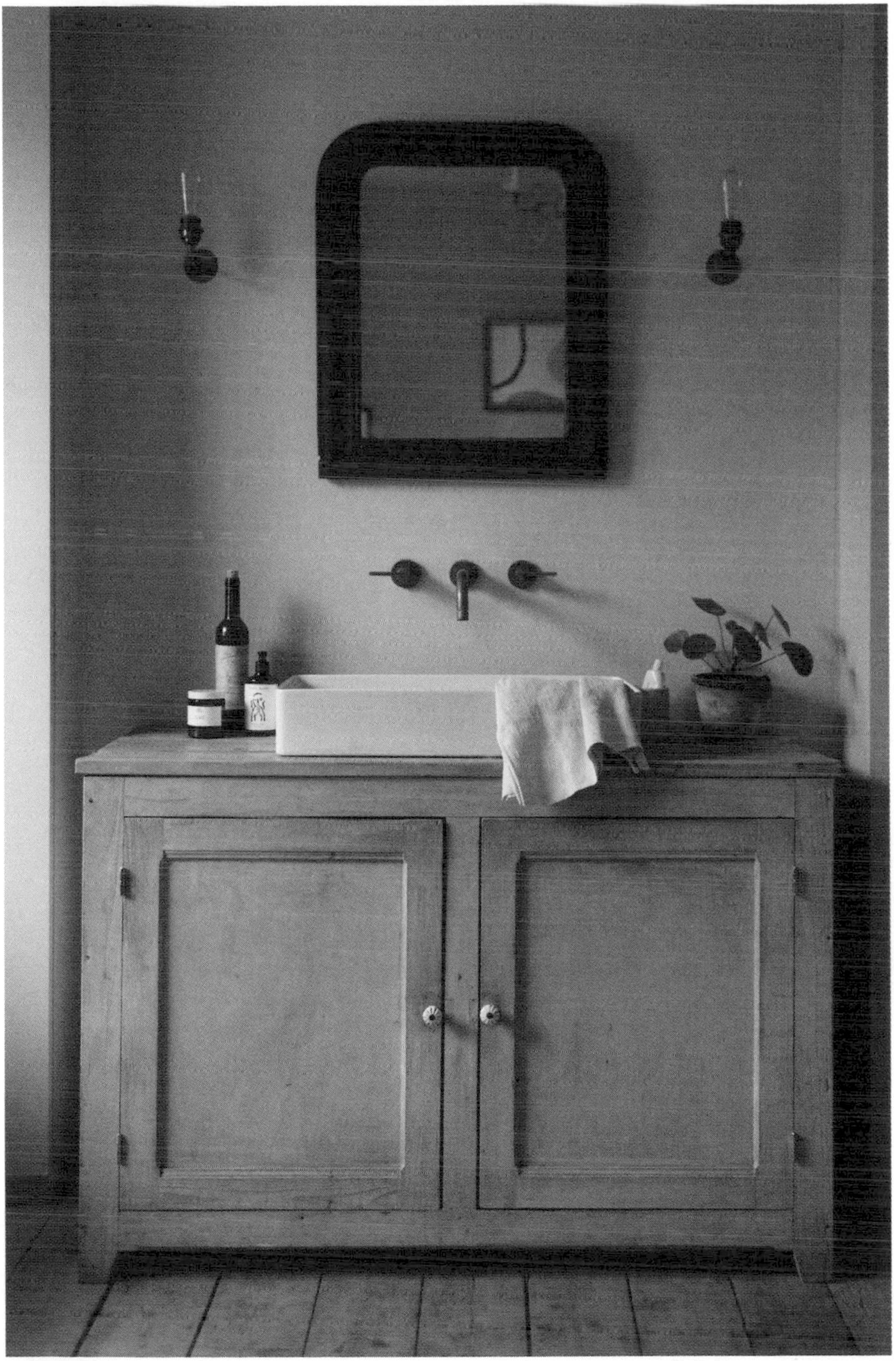

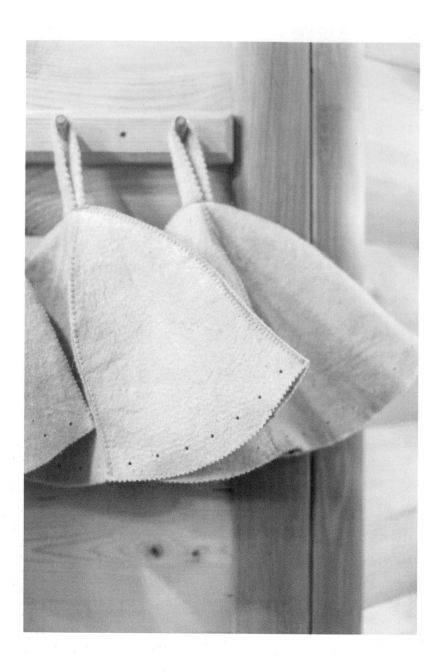

156   Bathe

No pain, no gain:
A guide to Russian Banyas

Banyas are saunas with a difference. One of Russia's oldest traditions, they are deeply ingrained in their culture and are credited with keeping their countrymen clean and healthy. There is a vast number of banyas, from traditional standalone huts in rural areas through to public stone mansions with palace-like interiors in cities.

While they are sometimes compared to saunas because the set-up is similar, banyas are different to their foreign counterparts. In saunas, the air is hot and dry, with no more than 5 to 10 per cent humidity, but in banyas, there is far higher humidity – around 60 to 70 per cent; Russians believe hot and dry air in saunas dries the throat and skin. They pay particular attention to the quality of the steam. Water is thrown onto stones heated to extreme temperatures behind metal doors, which creates steam droplets of an exceptionally small size. Sometimes a few drops of eucalyptus or pine oil are added to the water to create an aroma as the steam is released.

There are two types of banya: Classic black and modern white. Traditional black banyas have an open-flame stone stove in the centre of the room; the smoke goes out through the door or a special hole in the wall. The birch wood fire is surrounded by boulders, which heat the building; women traditionally gave birth here because it is a sterile environment. The white banya is the more modern version, where smoke goes through a chimney flue. Unless it's a family banya, men and women attend the bath at separate times.

Banyas consist of three rooms:

• **A predbannik**, where people get changed and leave their clothes.

- **A washing room** for visitors to wash prior to entering the banya.

- **The steam room** – parilka – where people go to bathe. All modern banyas have different layouts but most can accommodate several people.

Like saunas, banyas are about leisure time, relaxation and enjoyment. The idea is to start on the lower benches to get used to the temperature before moving up to the higher ones. Novices typically spend between five and seven minutes relaxing.

WOOD AND A WHIPPING –
THE RUSSIAN MASSAGE THAT IS
NOT FOR THE FAINT-HEARTED

As bathers get used to the temperatures, next comes the most indispensable part of the banya experience – the venik, a bunch of thin birch or oak branches, which are used to whip each other. One person lies down on his stomach and he is whipped before switching places with the other. Russians firmly believe in the power of this beating to enhance circulation, sweating and metabolism. The oils in venik leaves are said to improve the condition of the skin and have an anti-ageing effect.

This is then followed by a dip in an ice-cold bath or plunge pool. Russians believe the contrasting extremes of cold and heat are the key to achieving bliss. They then return to the parilka and repeat the routine several times, with breaks for tea.

Are we short-changing our bathtime?

You have had a long, hard day at work and are desperate to wash away the day's stresses. How long do you bathe for, or do you completely forsake the bath in favour of a hasty shower? The hectic pace of modern life means that time-saving showers are king in the UK. According to one poll, while the majority of people's houses contain baths, a third of Brits only take a bath four times a year. The average time people spend in the bath is around 20 minutes.

Try carving out time for a bath and give yourself the opportunity to enjoy it. After ten minutes of soaking you might be tempted to hop out and get on with something else. Fight the urge and lie back for at least another ten minutes. The products in the bath will need time to work their magic and it will greatly benefit your body and mind.

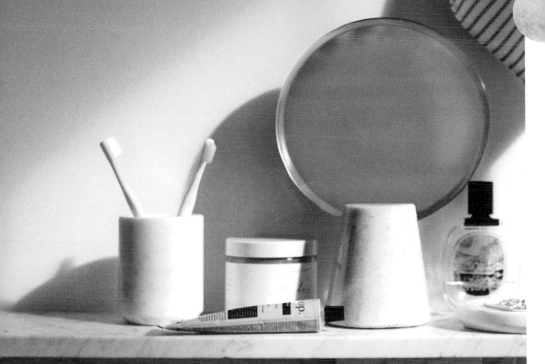

Jimjilbang: The South Korean one-stop shop to relaxation

South Korean saunas or spas give their visitors the gift of time and a 24/7 rotating door of group self-care where people shower, soak, steam, scrub and soothe in an endless stream. Translated as 'heated rooms', jimjilbang are an important part of contemporary South Korean culture and a newer version of the public bathhouses that were popularised during Japanese rule. As with onsen, these are large, gender-segregated bathhouses where everyone from young couples to grannies comes to hang out with their friends and family, relax, unwind and engage in a number of health and beauty rituals.

Visits here are not rushed affairs. Open 24 hours a day, jimjilbang are cheap to enter and a place where people can stay overnight. Many people travel with their families for weekend breaks to relax and revitalise, while some men will stay in jimjilbang overnight after an evening out with colleagues. Visitors are never clock-watching and there is no such thing as overstaying your welcome. Most basic entry fees give visitors 12 hours of unlimited use of the different baths and saunas.

In their modern incarnation, jimjilbang reflect South Korea's relatively new wealth, while also giving a nod to the public baths of old. They are furnished with baths and tubs featuring a mix of different herbal infusions and temperatures, wet and dry saunas, showers, common rooms with heated floors and massage tables. Most jimjilbang also feature snack bars, sleeping quarters, exercise rooms, cinemas, salt rooms, karaoke rooms and ice rooms. You can have a range of beauty treatments, haircuts and your shoes shined. Men and women bathe in separate baths but the saunas and other entertainment areas may be mixed.

Going to a jimjilbang is a personal and community experience. The communal nature of the buildings also suits many Koreans, who traditionally used to live with their extended families. There is a wonderfully welcoming atmosphere, genuinely no comparison between bodies and everyone's presence is valid.

'Many people travel with their families for weekend breaks to relax and revitalise, while some men will stay in jimjilbang overnight after an evening out with colleagues'

JIMJILBANGS: THE HOW-TO

Small groups: Visitors tend to go on their own or in groups of no more than about three people. Some people talk quietly and socialise while others relax in silence.

Get clean first: After entering the sex-segregated changing and shower rooms (usually on the first or second floor of the jimjilbang), strip off and shower. As in Japan, being completely naked is commonplace. Visitors always tie their hair up to be hygienic. Some people take their own toiletries or they are available to purchase.

Enjoy the baths: Guests then explore the varying temperatures of the pools and baths. Visitors regulate their body temperatures by cooling down in the showers regularly.

Scrub: After bathing, South Koreans give themselves and each other a firm scrub down using scrub mitts or this is performed by the 'scrub mistress'. They also shave, brush their teeth and can perform other personal care tasks, such as choosing to have a massage.

Dry fun: Once clothed in jimjilbang shorts and T-shirts, visitors can now enjoy the dry areas, which include fitness centres, snack bars, TV rooms and floor space for reading, relaxing or sleeping.

Sleep: All jimjilbang have communal sleeping rooms; some have bunks, while in others people sleep on ondol-heated floors (Korean heating system comprising hot water pipes under the floor) on a mat. Traditionally these pipes were heated with heat and smoke from the fire. Some jimjilbang sleeping rooms are gender-separated and some even have separate rooms for those who snore!

SESHIN AND THE SCRUB MISTRESS

The intense Korean body scrub (or seshin) is considered an essential part of the jimjilbang experience. All scrub mistresses will ask patrons to lie down naked on plastic beds before getting to work with a thin mitt with a sandpaper-like texture, scouring dead skin from the body. Afterwards, the body is rinsed with warm water and milk to soften and hydrate the skin. Some people may opt for a massage or another beauty treatment afterwards. From a Westerner's point of view, the experience is said to be awkward and uncomfortable (the scrub mistress leaves no part of the body alone), leaving rolls of grey, dead skin behind, which are rinsed off afterwards. However, the seshin is famed for boosting circulation, aiding with detoxification, relaxing the body, boosting energy levels and leaving the skin glowing and radiant.

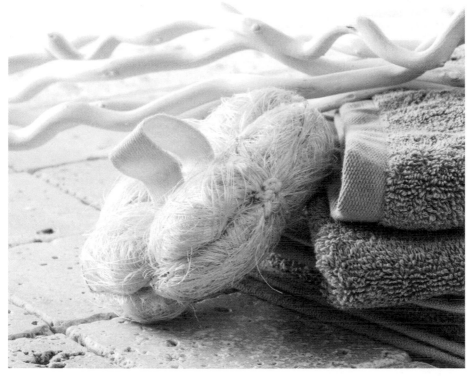

TOP TEN BATHING ACCESSORIES
AND WHY THEY MATTER

Choosing the right bathing accessories might make more difference than you may think and those little additions to your bathtime can have a big impact.

Bath tray: From rustic bamboo trays to stylish oak caddies, bath trays marry style and functionality and provide a handy place for resting other accessories.

Body brush: Dry brushing before the bath is a highly effective way of improving skin tone and stimulating blood and lymphatic circulation, kick-starting the metabolism and helping the body detoxify.

Muslin cloth: Muslins are a great way to remove cleansers to get that really deep-clean sensation.

Natural loofah: One of nature's best exfoliants, a loofah stays firm, while naturally exfoliating the body, improving circulation and skin condition.

Bath pillow: This is a lovely addition and cradles your head and cushions it, maximising both your comfort and safety.

Pumice stone: Using a cooled volcanic pumice stone, infused with minerals, is an excellent way to help remove dry skin and callouses.

Nail brush: Choose an elegantly curved brush that sits easily in your hand to cleanse both hands and nails.

Sea sponge: An all-natural alternative to washcloths, a sea sponge has a number of applications and they contain a multitude of minerals and enzymes to rejuvenate the skin.

Japanese wash cloth: A large textured cloth (usually nylon) that exfoliates is easier than a loofah to keep clean and helps produce an extra-creamy lather – an important step in the Japanese bathing ritual.

Moroccan hammam glove/mitt: This is used to deep cleanse, remove dead skin cells, toxins and impurities, and is often used with Beldi soap, made from black olive pulp.

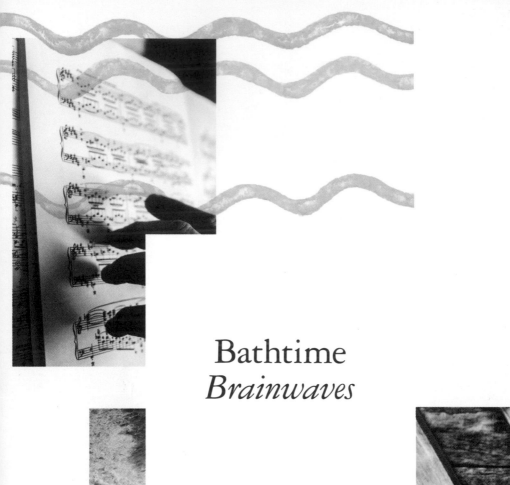

Bathtime
Brainwaves

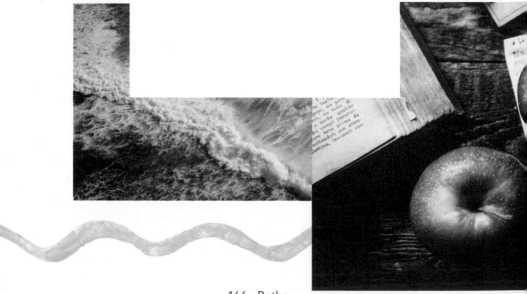

Here are two more famous faces who revelled in their daily dip and used it for creative inspiration.

[LUDWIG VAN BEETHOVEN]
1770-1827

The German composer is said to have found musical creativity and inspiration through bathing. He would stand at the washbasin and pour large pitchers of water over his hands and then walk up and down the bathroom, humming. Tenants living below the composer were said to complain regularly about the noise and leaks that would seep through the ceiling.

[AGATHA CHRISTIE]
1890-1976

The crime novelist and writer liked to dream up ideas while immersed in her large Victorian bath. She told her architect she wanted a big bath, with a ledge, so she could dream up new plots, while eating apples and drinking tea. Eventually she stopped the habit when she couldn't find baths that met her criteria. She claimed that modern baths were not built with authors in mind because they were 'too slippery with no nice wood ledge to rest pencils and paper on'.

RITUAL

Music to have on your bathtime playlist

When taking a long soak in the bath, it's not just the products you use that will help you unwind. It's been scientifically proven that calm music (classical, in particular) has a relaxing effect on the body and mind. Many streaming services like Spotify have their own bathtime playlists but if you would like a little inspiration to get you started, here are some ideas.

'The Long Day is Over' – Norah Jones
Unaccompanied cello suite No.1 In G Major – J.S. Bach
'Thinking Out Loud' – Ed Sheeran
'Liebestraum No. 3 in A Flat Major' – Franz Liszt
'Lay Me Down' – Sam Smith
'Songs Without Words' – Felix Mendelssohn
'You & I (Nobody in the World)' – John Legend
'"Raindrop" Preludes, Op 28, No. 15' – Frédéric Chopin
'How Long Will I Love You' – Ellie Goulding
'Canon in D Major' – Johann Pachelbel
'Moonlight Sonata' – Ludwig van Beethoven
'Last Request' – Paolo Nutini
'Clair de Lune' – Claude Debussy
'Love Is a Losing Game' – Amy Winehouse
'Largo (from "Xerxes")' – G.F. Handel
'Magic' – Coldplay
'Dancing On My Own' – Calum Scott
'I Like Myself' – Blossom Dearie

FIVE WAYS TO READ IN THE BATH

(WITHOUT GETTING YOUR BOOK WET!)

Reading a book while soaking in the bathtub is one of the simple joys in life but one question remains: how do you read without getting the pages wet? Here are some tips so your reading material stays dry at all times.

Get a bath tray: These trays lie across the width of the bath and will hold a book for you; some others may also have a special wineglass holder, so you can read with a glass of wine to hand.

Always have a dry towel nearby: In case you get your hands wet, keep a dry towel to hand, so you can dry them off to continue reading.

Use another stand: If you don't have a bath tray, you can improvise with a high stool or an old music stand. Prop your book up and give your hands a quick dry before turning the pages.

Choose a paperback: If you take your highly anticipated new hardback into the bath, chances are you won't be able to relax. Take an old paperback that may have been on your to-read list instead.

Listen to an audio book: This might not be quite the same as reading yourself but listening to an audio book (downloaded on a device out of arms reach!) read by one of your favourite authors or actors can really lift the spirits and brings the same intellectual benefits.

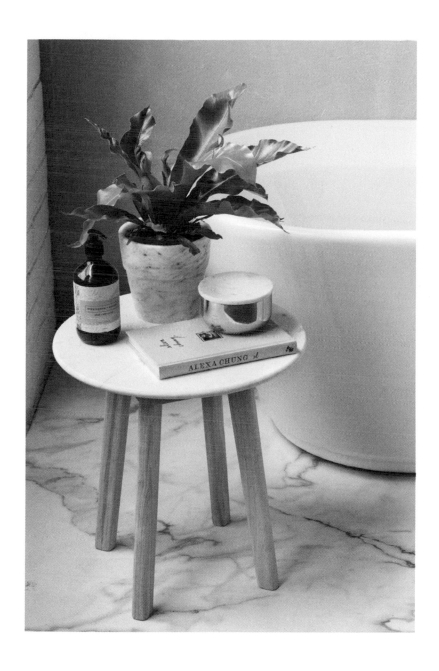

A guide to eating and drinking in the bath

A chilled glass of wine to sip while bathing gives a welcome hedonistic edge to self-care, aiding relaxation no end! It is never a good idea to bathe on a full stomach because this delays digestion as blood flows to other parts of the body. However, having nibbles and a hot or cold drink can bring a touch of indulgence.

Ideas could include grapes, apricots or a couple of squares of dark chocolate to eat or a small glass of red wine, an ice-cold, lime-infused gin and tonic or a small tumbler of whisky for refreshment. For the purists on the other hand, herbal teas make excellent bathing accompaniments: Burdock, red clover and milk thistle teas are excellent for aiding detoxing and cleansing; green tea, ginseng and black teas are energising; and peppermint, camomile and lemon palm teas are said to naturally help with anxiety and will leave you feeling serene.

RITUAL

'...having nibbles
and a hot or
cold drink can
bring a touch
of indulgence'

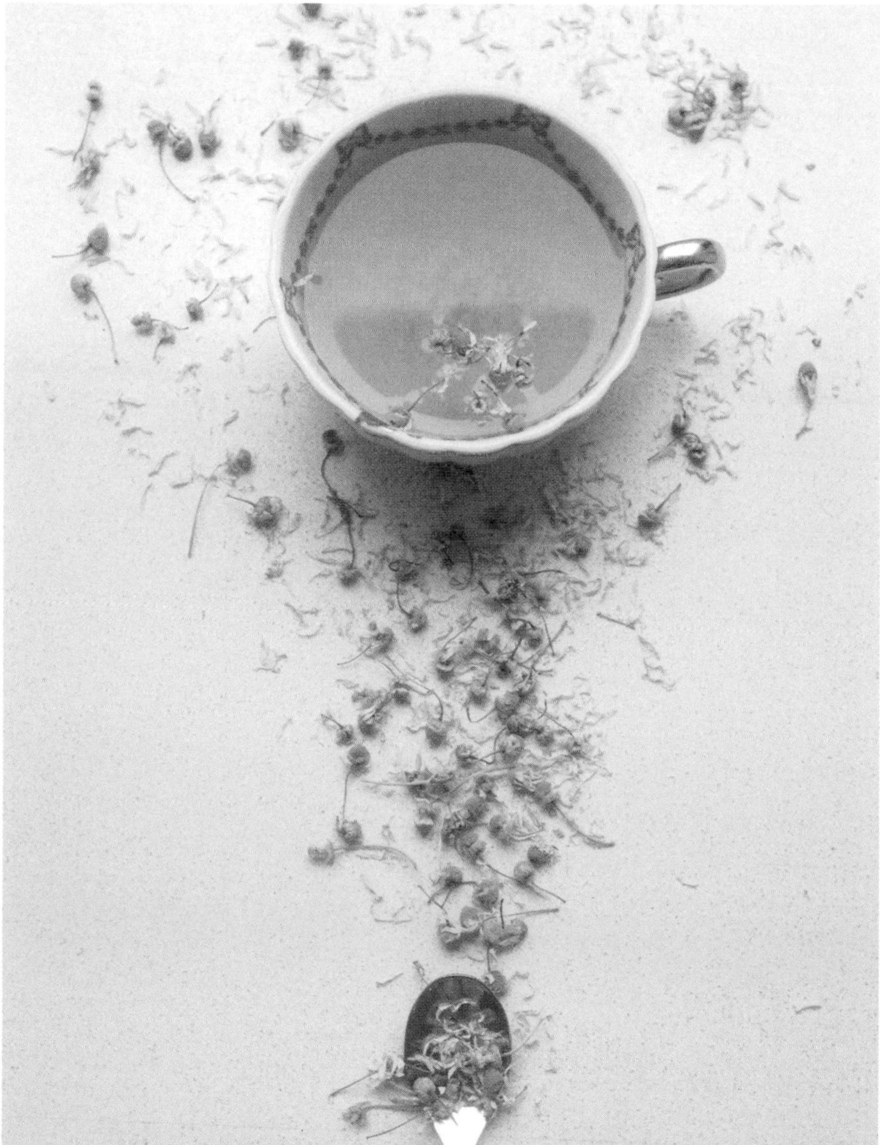

Clarity

'Water quiets all
the noise, all the
distractions, and
connects you to your
own thoughts'

[WALLACE J. NICHOLS]

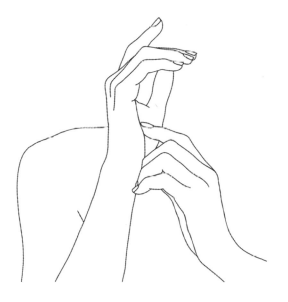

177 Bathe

The relaxing, solitary and non-judgemental act of bathing allows our minds to wander freely, this is a great catalyst for free association, where we can trigger ideas or revelations.

There have been many scientific studies into why we get these seemingly random insights, but far from being random, the relaxing, solitary and non-judgemental act of bathing allows our minds to wander freely. This is a great catalyst for free association, where we can trigger ideas or revelations. Switching into relaxation mode while you lie in the tub might be just what you need to coax out your inner genius! It is inexpensive and uncomplicated, yet potentially life-changing.

179 Bathe

The blue mind: Creativity and problem solving in the bath – why do we find clarity when bathing?

There is a peace and clarity that comes with being near water. We spend our holidays by a swimming pool or the sea, refresh ourselves with daily soothing showers and baths and many people dream of building their own homes and living near large expanses of water.

Our affinity with water is said to be reflected in our attraction to the colour blue. As well as the sea, blue is the colour of the clear sky and it is associated with open spaces, freedom, intuition, truth and depth. We are innately enticed by aquatic hues because they make our body and mind relax and exude feelings of tranquillity, order and calm. Time and again in research, blue is cited to be the world's favourite colour.

A US marine biologist, Wallace J. Nichols, who has dedicated his life to understanding the effects of water on our brains, believes we all have a 'blue mind' that is triggered when we are in or near water. Nichols describes this as a 'mildly meditative state characterised by calm, peacefulness, unity and a sense of general happiness and satisfaction with life at the moment'. He believes this calm state facilitates clarity and insight and allows us to tap into our most creative selves.

CLARITY

In our modern world, where we are hyper-stimulated and over-connected with technology, sitting too long at our desks and rushing against the clock and deadlines, we barely have time to breathe and take short, quick breaths. This is the opposite of what our bodies naturally crave: An existence where our minds can rest and wander freely. Being around water allows our brains and senses to rest from overstimulation; essentially, it is a holiday for our brains. We are constantly bombarded with sensory input and, like any muscle in our bodies, our brains need downtime; the sight and sound of water is much easier to process than any other information. People who float in water often register a change from more active brainwaves to slower theta brainwaves – brainwaves that reduce stress and aid healing. A relaxed state of mind is important to be creative; we release the hormone dopamine, which facilitates clarity and creativity.

When we relax, our brains switch into a different mode of engagement: A resting state, known as the default mode network. This is extremely important for creativity, and being in this state often allows us to solve problems by making new neural connections, unleashing a flow of creative ideas. You can see different situations from different perspectives. These ideas are widely considered to be some of the best problem-solving solutions our minds can generate.

'Being around water
allows our brains
and senses to rest
from overstimulation;
essentially, it is a
holiday for our brains'

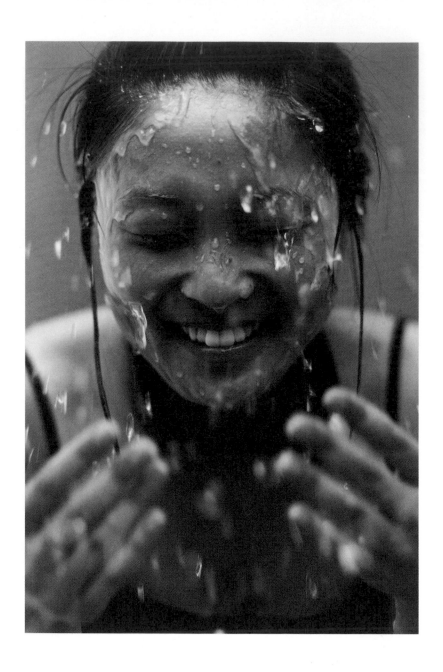

CLARITY

184   Bathe

FIVE BATHTIME EXERCISES TO

FUEL CREATIVE THINKING

Rarely do brilliant ideas just appear from nowhere. Creativity is not necessarily about coming up with new ideas but making connections between existing ones. If you want to tackle a difficult problem or simply want to challenge your creativity, next time you are in the bath, experiment with these strategies to make your next breakthrough:

Ask yourself: 'What else can I do with this?'. We see most objects, materials, spaces and technology through the lens of habit and familiarity, overlooking other possibilities. Asking yourself these questions may lead to new ideas and revelations.

Simplify it: Often the best ideas are the simplest ones and we over-complicate challenges due to an overload of information. Think about the challenge or problem you are facing and simplify it into 40 words, 20 words, ten words and then five words. Legend has it that Ernest Hemingway was challenged by other writers to compose a six-word story and he succeeded in writing a beginning, middle and end.

Make it personal: If you have a work problem, use aspects of your personal life to spark ideas – things you know about yourself or others in your personal life – and use this to analyse your work issue.

Go for quantity: Ask yourself how many solutions to a specific problem you can think of. Don't worry about quality and make it a game in your mind. This might just pave the way for some great ideas!

Make a wish: When thinking about a problem, think wishfully. This means you will move beyond sensible and practical ideas and are more likely to land on more original solutions through divergent thinking.

'Diplomacy without a tie': The Finnish art of networking in the nude

Finland loves its saunas – a top-to-toe immersion in dry heat. Here, it is completely normal to hold a business or political meeting in a sauna. With a population of 5.5 million people, there is one sauna for roughly every two people and most companies have an in-house sauna. It is not so much a luxury as an essential daily experience. Unlike in some other countries, the saunas here are single sex, but for non-Finnish newcomers, the first sessions in the cabin without a stitch of clothing might take some time to get used to!

The Finns believe that due to its social nature and relaxing effect, the sauna is an excellent place for exchanging opinions, brainstorming ideas and negotiations. Getting naked and talking about politics is also commonplace. All Finnish embassies, consulates and residencies have their own saunas. No one is allowed to argue; everyone is seen as equal and everyone must come out as friends. Urho Kekkonen, who governed for almost 26 years as the President of Finland during the Cold War, and Martti Ahtisaari, former president and Nobel Peace Prize laureate of 2008, held negotiations with foreign diplomats in the sauna. The method was dubbed 'diplomacy without a tie'.

According to reports, when the Soviet Premier Nikita Khrushchev came to Finland for Kekkonen's 60th birthday, they partied in the sauna until 5a.m. Soon after, the Soviets supported Finland's desire to integrate with the West. Finland's then Secretary of State explained: 'Decisions and negotiations take less time in the high heat. The sauna cools down overexcitement and melts away political differences.'

Inviting guests to the sauna is an old Finnish offering of hospitality and the Finns like to uphold this tradition when living abroad, where possible. At the Finnish Embassy in Washington DC, the monthly 150 member-strong Diplomatic Sauna Society sees Capitol Hill staffers, journalists, lobbyists and think-tankers network together once a month, with invitations extended to high-ranking politicians, such as former Vice President Joe Biden, who used to reside opposite the Embassy. Sauna diplomacy is said to go a long way towards calming and building relationships.

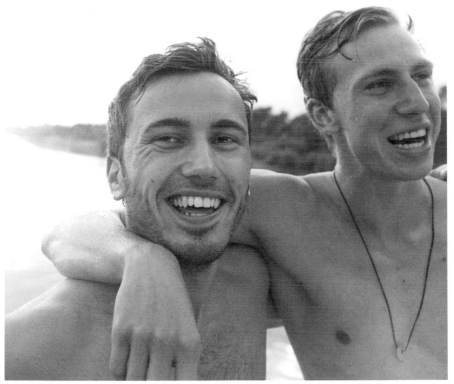

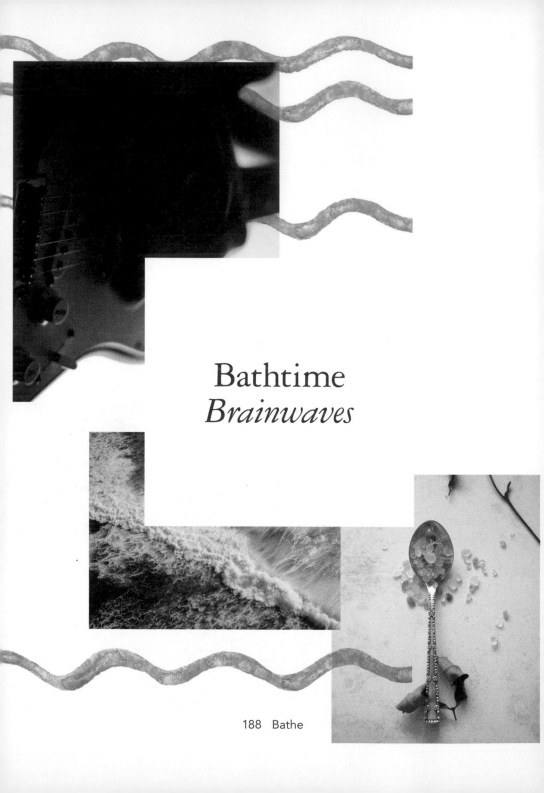

Bathtime
Brainwaves

Here are two more celebrated
personalities who love their soaks:

[FREDDIE MERCURY]
1946-1991

The lead singer of Queen wrote 'Crazy Little
Thing Called Love' while taking a bubble bath
in a hotel room in Munich. He got out of the
bath, wrapped a towel around himself and began
working on the chords there and then.

[ARIANNA HUFFINGTON]
1950-

The billionaire businesswoman and founder
of *The Huffington Post* takes a nightly bath before
bed with Epsom salts and candles. If she is feeling
anxious or stressed, she stays in the bath for longer.
'It's my ritual to wash away the day,' she says.

CLARITY

WHITE

Lars Müller Publishers   rs Müller Publishers

LONDON

CEREAL 12

CEREAL 11

Digital detoxing:
Technology has no place
in the bathroom!

Laptops in bed and smartphones in the bath... it's no wonder we struggle to switch off. Many of us have become slaves to our devices, with research showing that British adults spend more than eight hours per day on screens – more time than we spend asleep. We check our phones 10,000 times per year and recent scientific studies have proved that this makes us tired, anxious and more prone to depression and other mental health conditions.

Our tech habits keep us on high alert and greedy for more information to consume, denying our brains crucial downtime. The brain needs time and space to wander freely, think deeply, reflect and refocus. Also, numerous scientific studies show that the artificial blue light emitted from devices stops us from getting enough rest. Bathing provides another opportunity within our daily lives to unplug, be truly present in the moment and realise all is well, right here, right now.

CLARITY

A SIMPLE BATHTIME BREATHING EXERCISE

TO FEEL ENERGISED AND FOCUSED

Consider bathtime a great moment for washing and cleansing your mind as well as your body. The alternate nostril breathing technique – known to yogis as 'Nadi shodhana' – is simple and effective and ideal for practising in the bath. 'Nadi' is a Sanskrit word meaning channel or flow, while 'shodhana' means purification. The right side of the brain is said to be responsible for processing our emotions and influences our creativity, while the left side governs language and logic. This breathing practice is said to balance both sides of the brain, lowering tension and revitalising a tired mind and body, improving fine motor control.

Relax in the bath comfortably. Rest your left palm on your left knee.

Bring your right hand to your nose, then using your right thumb, close the right nostril and inhale as slowly as you can through your left nostril, then close it with your ring finger. Pause, release your thumb and exhale slowly through your right nostril.

With your right nostril open, inhale slowly, then close it with your thumb. Pause and release your ring finger, exhaling through the left nostril.

Inhale through the left nostril and pause before moving to the right.

Repeat this pattern five to ten times and then relax both arms and breathe normally.

'This breathing practice is said to balance both sides of the brain, lowering tension and revitalising a tired mind and body, improving fine motor control'

Shinrin-Yoku: The art of bathing in the forest

'The clearest way into the Universe
is through a forest wilderness'

[John Muir]

Shinrin-Yoku or 'forest bathing' is a Japanese practice of contemplative walking in the forest and soaking up the sights, sounds and smells of the natural setting. Developed in the 1980s, Shinrin-Yoku has become a cornerstone of preventative healthcare and healing in Japanese medicine. It draws on thousands of years of intuitive knowledge, providing a powerful antidote to modern life and helps us create a profound connection with nature.

Scientists in Japan have done a great deal of research into Shinrin-Yoku and its benefits, and have proved that spending time in the forest has a positive and calming effect on our bodies and minds. Benefits include a reduction of the stress hormone cortisol, lower blood pressure and heart rate, accelerated recovery from trauma or illness and improved overall feelings of well-being. Studies in other countries, including the US and Finland, have shown similar decreases in tension and anxiety.

Trees and plants emit phytoncides, antimicrobial organic compounds, which we breathe in when we're in the forest, that are said to boost our immune systems. One study showed that men who took two-hour walks in the forest over two days had a 50 per cent spike in natural killer cells, which are critical to our immune systems because they help our bodies fight disease. Women who logged four hours in the forest on two consecutive days also saw nearly a 40 per cent surge in the activity of cancer-fighting white blood cells. Another American study also showed that participants had a 50 per cent improvement in creative problem-solving after three days immersed in nature without access to technology. The meditative nature of being in the forest releases us from the distractions of modern life and allows our brains to be free and re-set. Combined with this are the well-established benefits of being outdoors within nature, such as improved sleep and more energy.

The exact mechanisms of Shinrin-Yoku remain unknown but there are now a vast number of accredited Shinrin-Yoku forests in Japan, conducting research and aiming at establishing forest therapy around the world. If you are a city-dweller, a simple dose of nature could improve your physical health and well-being.

SOUL–CLEANSING: HOW TO BATHE
WELL IN THE FOREST

Like bathing in water, bathing in the forest is not a competition. It is a personal experience, accessible to everyone, and fulfils an intrinsic yearning to reconnect with nature, of which we are a major part.

The practice is a technology-free one, so you must leave your phone, camera and any other distractions behind, to allow yourself to be present.

The intention of Shinrin-Yoku is to connect with nature. It requires walkers to be mindful, noticing and appreciating the forest. Feel the dense heaviness of the mud or leaves beneath your feet, listen to the sweet sound of birdsong and admire the delicate and intricate colours of the leaves, branches and plants.

You can wander aimlessly, take time to stand still or sit and observe nature around you. If you are walking with someone else, resist the urge to talk.

Shinrin-Yoku is not a rushed affair and its primary goal is not exercise but to inspire awe and wonder. This is a fantastic way to increase our depth of experience and understanding of the world around us.

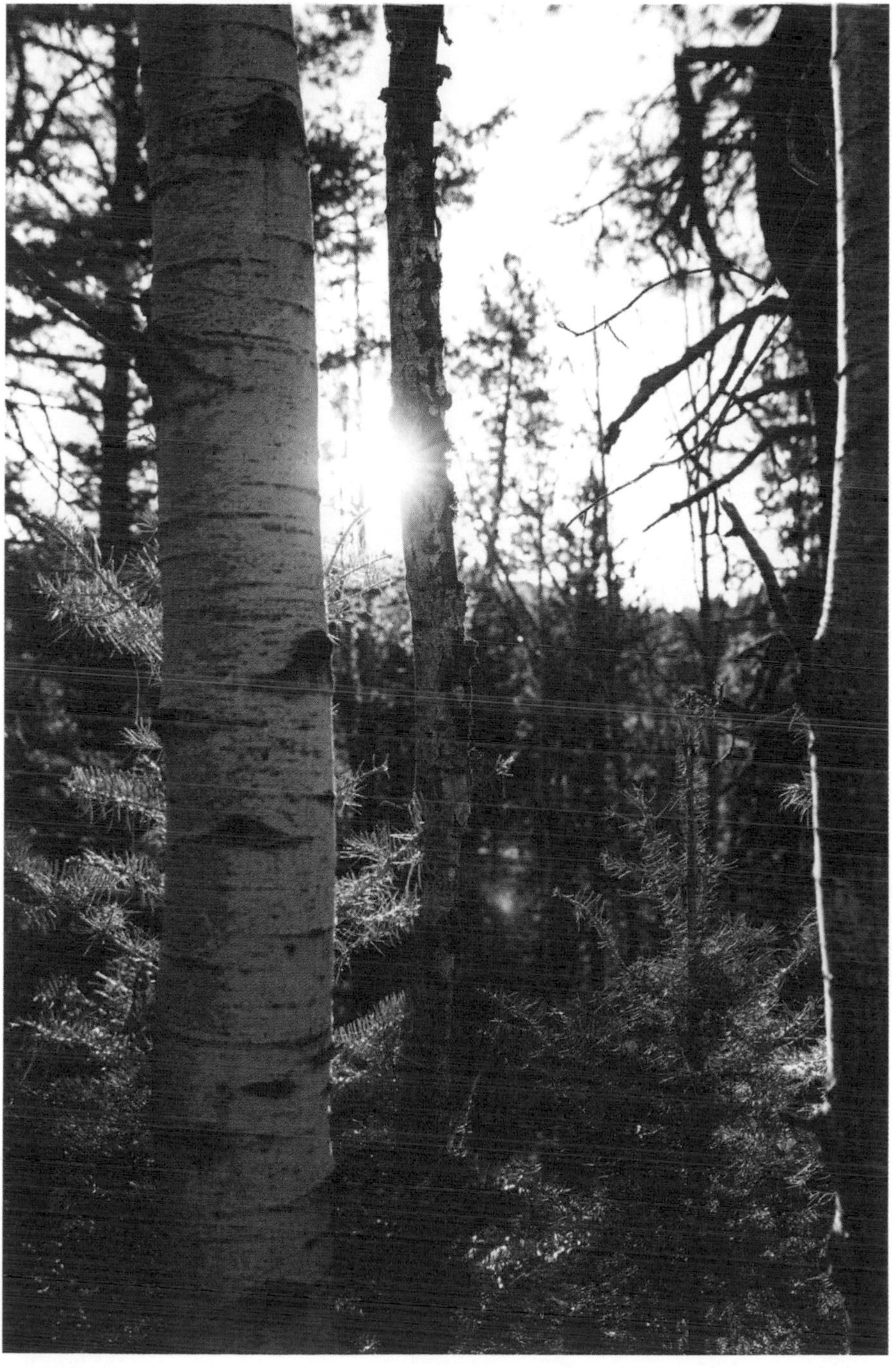

Romantic poetry and an encounter with the sublime

The British have long enjoyed a love affair with wild water swimming and wild bathing. Bathing and swimming feature in literature, art and music from the earliest days. For the British Romantic poets, wild bathing and swimming held a specific importance. This intellectual movement that originated towards the end of the 18th century in Europe saw nature as the most sublime phenomenon, capable of generating profound feelings of awe, ecstasy or reverence; emotions that almost transcend rational thought, words or language. Romantic poets went bathing and swimming in the sea, rivers and lakes, convinced that communing with nature would inspire their work.

William Wordsworth bathed in Derwentwater in Cumbria as a child, his experience informing his sense of connectedness with nature. Percy Bysshe Shelley was irresistibly drawn to the water and mesmerised by its mystical properties, bathing whenever he got the chance. He never learned to swim and eventually drowned, aged 29, in the Bay of Spezia in Northern Italy when his boat went down in a sudden storm. Lord Byron was a dramatic, daring and brave swimmer, jumping into Venetian canals and swimming away from romantic entanglements. He felt his sporting achievements were far superior to anything he achieved in his writing and sought to make wild swimming bohemian and enigmatic.

Samuel Taylor Coleridge gives an account of sea bathing in his lesser-known poem, 'On Revisiting the Sea-Shore, After Long Absence'. First published in the *Morning Post* in 1802, Coleridge had been suffering ill health and instead of using salt water baths, as advised by his physician, he plunged into the sea. He wrote in a letter: 'I bathed regularly, frolicked in the Billows and it did me a proper deal of good.'

Contemporary wild swimming and bathing is beholden to Romanticism. Wild bathers believe today, as they did then, that cold water is a time-honoured cure for depression and promotes superior physical health, as well as sparking joy and creativity.

199 Bathe

'On Revisiting the Sea-
Shore, After Long Absence'
by Samuel Taylor Coleridge

God be with thee, gladsome Ocean!
How gladly greet I thee once more!
Ships and waves, and ceaseless motion,
And men rejoicing on thy shore.

Dissuading spake the mild physician,
'Those briny waves for thee are Death!'
But my soul fulfill'd her mission,
And lo! I breathe untroubled breath!

Fashion's pining sons and daughters,
That seek the crowd they seem to fly,
Trembling they approach thy waters;
And what cares Nature, if they die?

Me a thousand hopes and pleasures,
A thousand recollections bland,
Thoughts sublime, and stately measures,
Revisit on thy echoing strand:

Dreams, (the Soul herself forsaking),
Tearful raptures, boyish mirth;
Silent adorations, making
A bless'd shadow of this Earth!

O ye hopes that stir within me,
Health comes with you from above!
God is with me, God is in me!
I cannot die, if Life be Love.

Calm

'In one drop of water
are found all the secrets
of all the oceans'

[KHALIL GIBRAN]

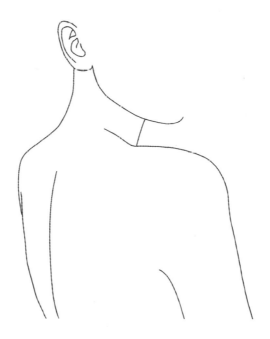

205 Bathe

Baths are innately unhurried,
contemplative and gentle.

CALM

A natural way to detox from digital devices, they
have evolved from a way of getting clean to getting
calm by providing a window of tranquillity to unwind
from the daily stresses of modern living.

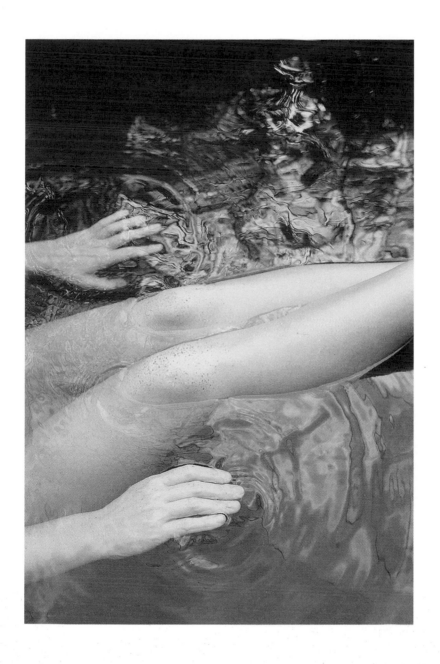

207 Bathe

THREE DIY BATH RECIPES TO SOOTHE, CALM AND BEAUTIFY THE SKIN

The key to maximising our time in the bath is using the right ingredients. When we love bathing, it might be tempting to spend every penny on expensive bath products, but before you draw your next bath, here are some rejuvenating and healing recipe ideas made from ingredients you probably have at home in your kitchen cupboard.

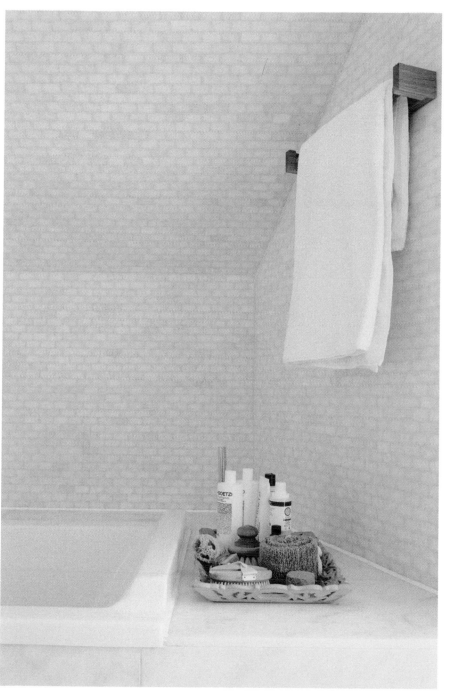

CALM

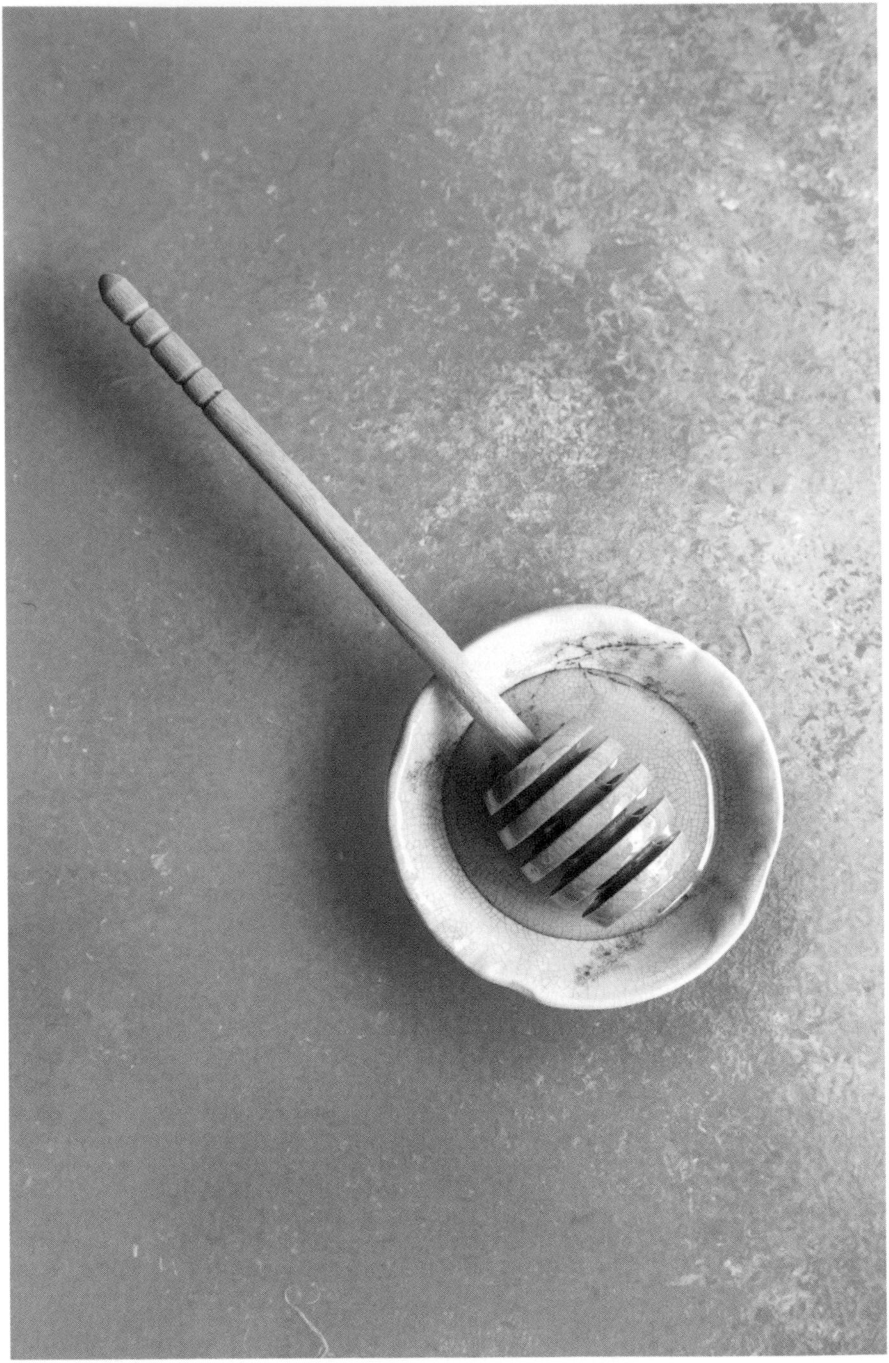

Oatmeal and Honey

If you are a fan of porridge for breakfast, you are probably already aware of the naturally nourishing benefits of oats. They can be the perfect ingredient to add to your bath, especially during winter. Oats provide soothing relief for dry skin, rashes, sunburn and everyday skin irritation. They also contain natural cleansers that help skin maintain its natural moisture barrier and keep pores free of impurities. Raw honey is also known to simultaneously cleanse and hydrate the skin.

How to use it: Add one to two cups (240ml to 475ml) of uncooked oats and let them stand in hot water and half a cup of honey for five minutes, then transfer the mixture to a muslin cloth or popsock to hold it together and avoid bunging up the plughole when you let the water out. Tie under a running tap and rest in the bath for at least 20 minutes afterwards.

CALM

Coconut Oil

This wonder oil has antibacterial, anti-inflammatory and antifungal benefits and encourages supple skin, softening it and even healing minor damage. It is loaded with good fats and is a natural source of vitamin E, a powerful antioxidant commonly found in anti-ageing skincare.

How to use it: Create a simple detox bath with coconut oil by adding a quarter of a cup of Epsom salts to a quarter of a cup (60ml) of coconut oil into a hot bath.

For an exfoliating bath, add half a cup (120ml) of coconut oil and half a cup (100g) of sugar to make a DIY body scrub.

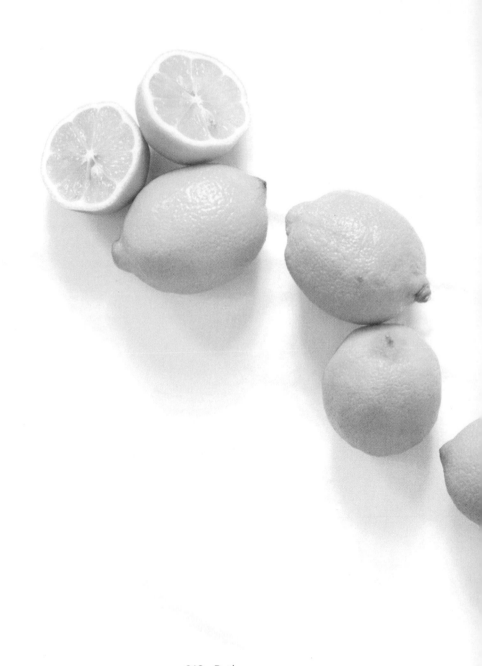

Ginger and Fresh Lemon Juice

Ginger has amazing antibacterial and anti-inflammatory properties, so this is ideal if you are fighting a cold or are congested. It is also warming, so will encourage your body to rid itself of toxins through sweating, leaving you zingy and glowing from top to toe. Lemon juice is rich in antioxidants and vitamin C, and will leave your skin looking refreshed.

How to use it: Add half a cup (120ml) of fresh lemon juice and either half a cup (145g) of grated ginger or ginger powder to a hot or warm bath. Rest in the bath for at least 20 minutes.

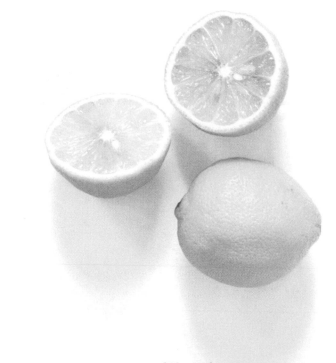

CALM

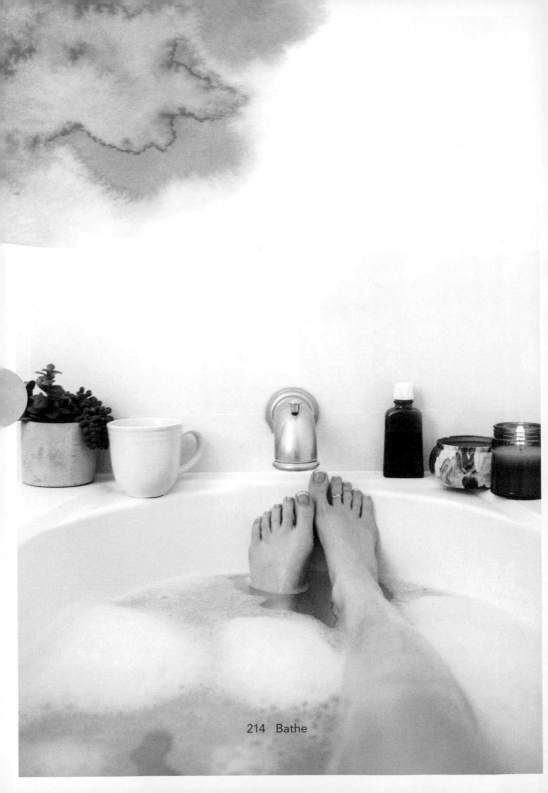

A bath before bedtime:
Why is a bath the perfect
wind-down activity?

We bathe children before they go to sleep and everyone cites this
as an essential part of a pre-bedtime routine. Why? Taking a hot bath
before bed induces sleep because your body temperature plays a big
part in how quickly you fall asleep. At night, there is a slight drop in
our body temperature, which signals to our bodies to start producing
melatonin, the hormone that induces sleep.

Having a bath raises our body temperature artificially before allowing
it to drop again, as you adjust to the cooler environment of the bedroom.
It is important to take a bath an hour or two before bed and make the
temperature warm rather than hot, so you are comfortable and your
body can gently cool down in the run-up to bedtime.

Alternatively, if you do not wish to take a full bath at night, studies
have shown that a simple footbath, simply sitting with your feet in hot
water can also help you relax and improves your sleep quality.

CALM

Aromatherapy: Natural healing through bathing

'The way to health is to have an aromatic
bath and scented massage every day'

[Hippocrates]

Aromatherapy is a holistic therapy that treats the body, mind and spirit and smells absolutely divine. Aromatherapy essential oils are created using hundreds of medicinal flowers, plants, herbs, trees and roots grown all around the world, which have proven and powerful effects on improving well-being. Aromatherapy is said to treat the whole person and not just the symptom or disease by assisting the body's natural ability to balance, regulate, heal and maintain itself.

Aromatherapy has a long history, as early as 3,000 BC, where the ancient Egyptians used scented ointments to beautify their hair, skin and nails. The use of aromatic medicines was also prolific in Ancient Greece and Rome. Indian and Chinese cultures also have long histories of using plant oils as medicine. In 1937, the first book about aromatherapy was written by French chemist René-Maurice Gattefossé, who worked with essential oils.

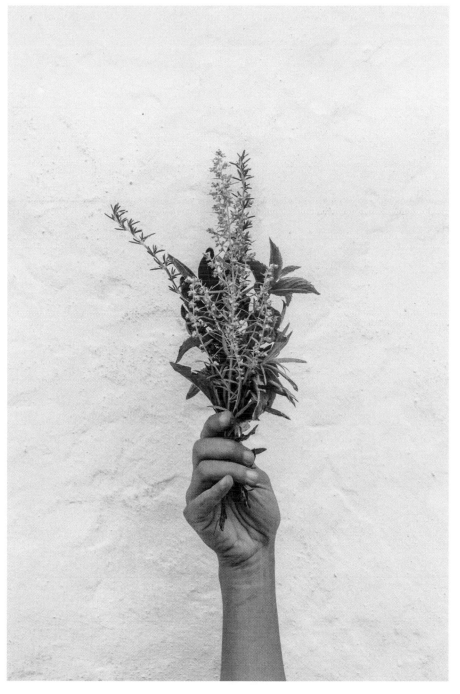

HOW DOES AROMATHERAPY WORK?

Bathing and aromatherapy have a clear synergy because baths give the oils a double route into the body: Through inhalation of the scent diffused in the steam and through the skin. When essential oils are absorbed through the body or inhaled, they can rejuvenate, invigorate tired bodies, boost circulation, promote detoxing, stimulate the immune system, relieve stress and lift mood. How this happens is the result of a complex process within the limbic system, an area of the brain associated with smell and memory.

The sense of smell is the most primitive and powerful of all our senses and is linked to some of the deepest parts of the brain. The olfactory nerves, located in the front of the brain, are responsible for sending signals about what we smell through the limbic system, which is commonly referred to as 'the emotional brain'. This information is then compared with our memory and emotional responses to that smell. It is said that our bodies can process thousands of different smells and remember them. The response to the smell then triggers a number of chemical actions within the body, related to heart rate, blood pressure, stress levels and hormone balance.

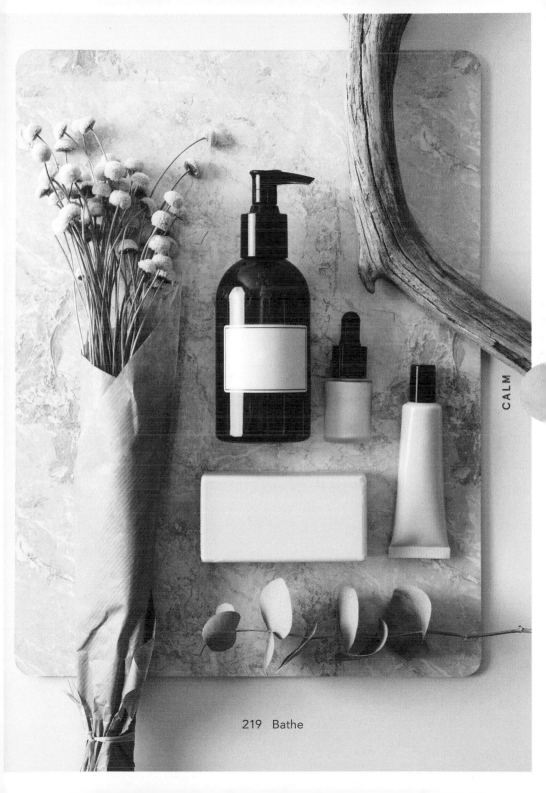

CALM

219 Bathe

'South Korean research
found that lavender
had a beneficial effect
on insomnia and
depression in women
college students'

WHY IS AROMATHERAPY SO POPULAR?

Today, aromatherapy is one of the most popular complementary medicines. It offers a wide range of effective treatments for a number of illnesses and there are many notable studies on the subject. One study found that the essential oil jasmine can lift mood and counteract symptoms of depression, while South Korean research found that lavender had a beneficial effect on insomnia and depression in women college students. It has also been proven that aromatherapy can aid sleep; one study found that essential oils placed nightly on towels around the pillows of patients suffering with dementia resulted in significantly longer sleep time, increased sustained sleep and reduced early morning waking. Another study looked at the effects of the inhalation of lavender oil on vital signs of patients during heart surgery and found that it led to significant reductions in blood pressure and heart rate.

CALM

SIX HEALING AROMATHERAPY
BATH RULES

Use a carrier oil: The safest and most effective way to use essential oils in the bath is to mix them with a carrier oil. Popular examples of carrier oils include almond oil and jojoba oil, which will allow the essential oils to disperse well and have the added benefit of moisturising and conditioning the skin.

Discard old oils: Like all products, essential oils have expiration dates and some oils will last longer than others. Keep them in a cool, dark place and if you notice an oil smells like it has gone off, discard it.

Do not skimp on quality: The purer the oil, the greater the benefits compared to the cheap and cheerful alternatives. Buy organic oils that are distilled or cold-pressed, which smell incredible.

Test first: Some oils can cause sensitisation so 48 hours prior to using an essential oil for the first time, perform a skin patch test using a couple of drops of diluted essential oil. Never use essential oils undiluted on the skin.

Avoid when pregnant: While some essential oils may be safe to use when pregnant, others can cause complications, so always check with a doctor before using essential oils when pregnant or nursing.

Use sparingly: Essential oils can be powerful, so never exceed the recommended dosage for use. Start by using any essential oil in minimal doses before increasing to get the results you desire.

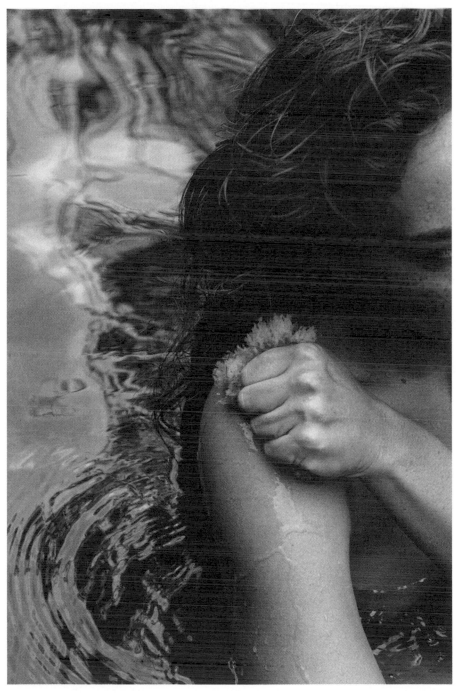

TWENTY HEALING NATURAL INGREDIENTS
AND HOW THEY COULD HELP YOU

Lavender: Well known for its calming and soothing properties, lavender is said to improve stress, aid sleep and help to heal burns, cuts, stings and other wounds.

Frankincense: This is often used to treat issues related to digestion, respiratory concerns and stress. It is also reputed to have anti-inflammatory properties and can boost the immune system.

Lemon: Citrus essential oils are said to stimulate circulation and lymph drainage. Lemon is also thought to have purifying, cleansing and uplifting properties on the mind and body.

Rosemary: Rosemary essential oil is said to aid digestion, and improve circulation and cognitive function.

Sandalwood: Antiseptic and soothing, sandalwood softens and protects the skin. It is also said that it can help users achieve greater clarity and calm.

Tea tree: Anti-viral, anti-bacterial and anti-fungal, tea tree oil can be used to treat cuts, infections, insect bites and even dandruff. It is also recognised as a powerful acne treatment.

Eucalyptus: This is an anti-viral, anti-bacterial and anti-spasmodic oil, used for coughs and colds and to aid the lymphatic system. It also refreshes and calms the skin.

Roman camomile: This is known for its ability to help unwind, encouraging soothing and comforting emotions. Gentler than tea tree oil, it is said to promote smooth and healthy skin.

Clary sage: This oil helps to calm the nervous system, lowering blood pressure and breathing rates. It is also said to be a natural pain killer and can help relieve headaches, back pain and muscle cramps.

Peppermint: This is another powerful oil, which is said to help with digestive issues and tight muscles. It also helps improve mental focus and boosts energy.

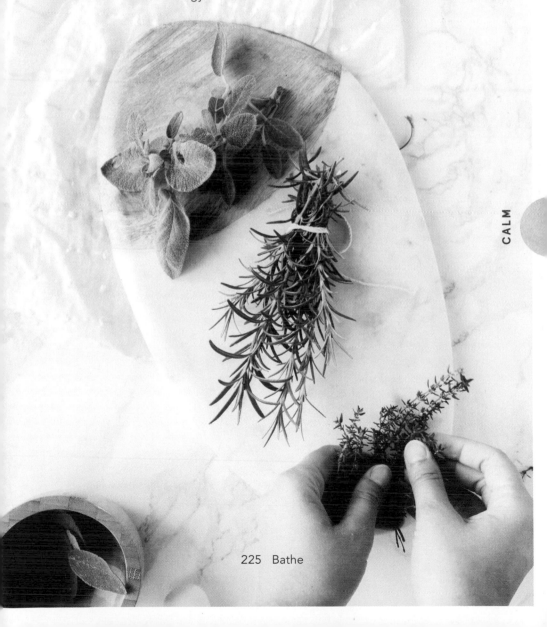

Neroli: This is said to calm the body and mind and balance the skin. It also helps to alleviate digestive issues.

Grapefruit: This oil helps to boost circulation and is a natural digestive aid. The invigorating aroma also increases energy.

Bergamot: With its powerful aroma, this fresh essential oil improves circulation and is said to help cure ailments associated with stress, such as insomnia and high blood pressure.

Aloe vera: Like aloe vera gel, aloe vera oil is known for its ability to promote skin health, help heal sunburn and can ease other skin conditions, like eczema.

Ylang ylang: This oil is said to have an uplifting effect on mood and is effective at treating high blood pressure. It also promotes healthy hair and skin.

Geranium: Geranium helps to harmonise the body and balance hormones. It also improves circulation and minimises inflammation.

Patchouli: Naturally anti-fungal and anti-inflammatory, patchouli also has a reputation for being a grounding and soothing oil.

Bay: This oil warms and comforts the body and mind and can help relieve muscle pain and discomfort. It is also said to be a natural decongestant and can ease respiratory infections.

Cardamom: Fortifying and invigorating, cardamom is believed to reduce drowsiness and improve concentration. It is also a natural antiseptic.

Pine: Known for clearing the mind and helping to energise the body, pine is also said to boost the immune system and reduce inflammation.

CALM

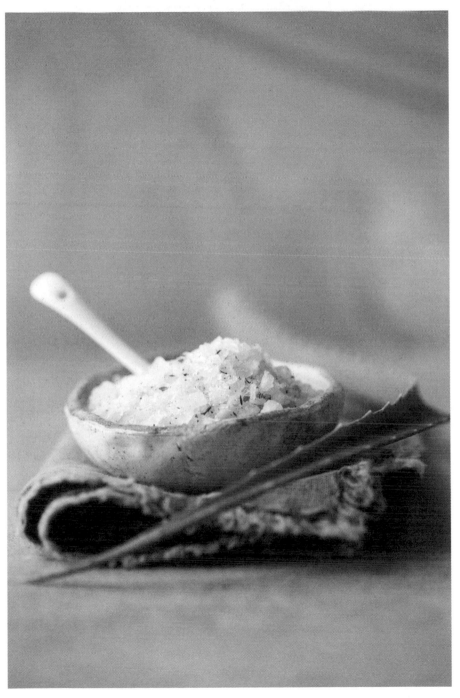

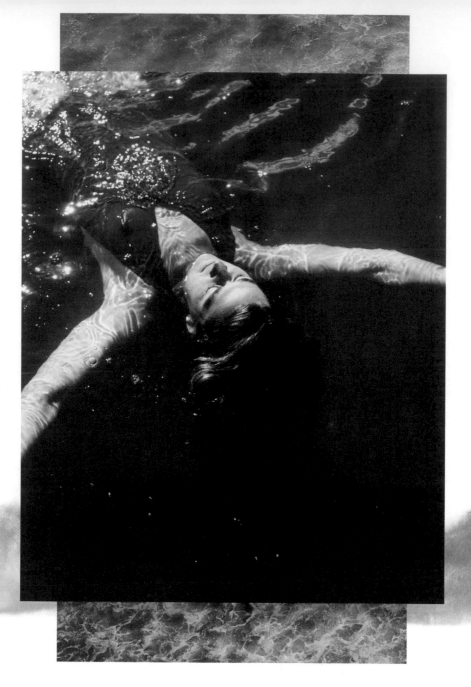

228 Bathe

Weightless:
Discover the hidden
joys of flotation

Flotation therapy is the practice of lying down in a flotation tank and drifting into a deep meditative state. The water is infused with magnesium-rich Epsom salts, creating an environment that is similar to the Dead Sea, but air and skin temperatures are controlled in the tank, so they are the same. This allows a feeling of weightlessness and the pods are designed to block out all noises and external distractions.

Flotation therapy promotes calmness and relaxation by alleviating both physical and mental stress; it eliminates fatigue, improves sleep, increases mental clarity and motivation, boosts circulation, relieves pain and improves athletic performance.

CALM

CALM

Gong baths –
What are they?

If you want another calming and healing way of bathing, rather than submerging yourself in water, consider immersing yourself in sound waves. A gong bath is a form of sound therapy where a gong is played in a therapeutic way to bring about healing; this can be done on a one-to-one basis or in a group setting. This form of sound therapy goes back thousands of years. The ancient Asian technique, where participants are 'bathed' in sound waves, is said to produce an amazing feeling of well-being through the vibration of water within the body. The therapy is thought to heal the resting nervous system, aid stress reduction and break emotional blockages and can be used to manage a variety of health conditions.

While there is little scientific research into gong baths and sound healing, anecdotal evidence is strong and there are many studies citing the profound ways that music affects the brain. Some studies have shown patients who are exposed to music report less pain, while large-scale reviews of over 400 research papers into the neurochemistry of music show that listening to music has clear benefits for mental and physical health.

CALM

Take a moment: Relaxation after the bath

Bathtime is a relaxing ritual, but time spent after the bath needs to be given the same level of attention and care. In Japan, this moment is known as 'Yuagari', which translates as 'the moment after the bath'. This is a moment of luxuriant tranquillity during which your body cools down. Sip tea or another refreshing drink, let your body relax and allow yourself to be idle before you continue with your day.

'This is a moment of luxuriant tranquillity during which your body cools down'

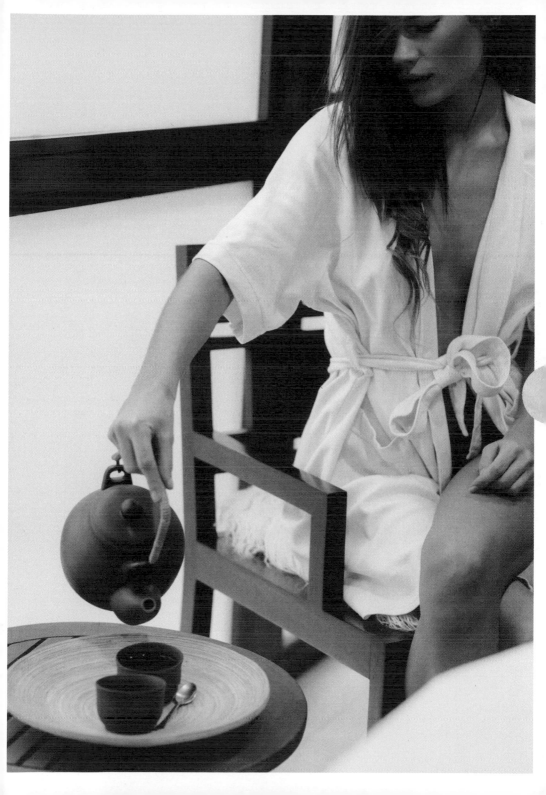

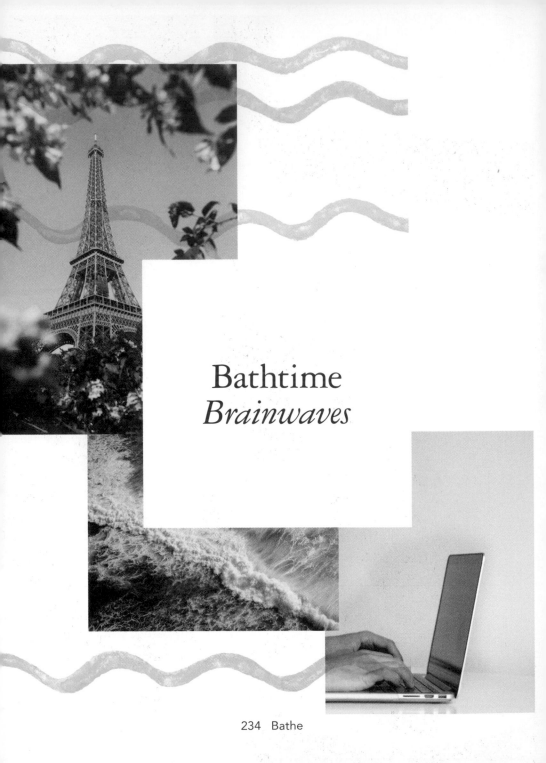

Bathtime
Brainwaves

Baths have always been seen by many well-known figures as a place to rest, recharge and tackle their work.

[VICTOR HUGO]
1802–1885

The French writer and author of *Les Misérables* had quite a unique daily morning routine. It would start with two raw eggs and a coffee before he took a two-hour ice-cold public bath on the roof of his home, with the water left out overnight, to get him in the creative mood.

CALM

[TOM FORD]
1961–

The filmmaker and fashion designer is a big fan of meditative baths and has up to five baths a day to help calm him when he is busy and stressed. 'If I'm sending emails and I get all wound up and stressed and don't know what to do with myself for 20 minutes,' he says, 'I just go soak in hot water and sit there thinking, "What should I do?" It's so meditative.'

Raising the bar:
The simple soap

Time to dust down your soap dish! Once skin-stripping bricks, the quality and formulae of soap bars have improved drastically over recent years and sophisticated formulae are making them more 'beauty bars' than humble soaps. There are now soaps for every beauty need, from body-buffing through to skin-soothing, and most are very affordable and beautifully packaged. Here are a few variations worth getting in a lather over!

MOROCCAN BLACK SOAP

Named after its colour, this soap was originally made in Syria using vegetable soda and olive oil, before migrating to Morocco. The basic recipe remains the same but now includes essential oils and is a key part of the Moroccan hammam ritual. This soap is gently cleansing and is good for various skin conditions, like rosacea and eczema.

SUPERFATTED SOAP

These are normal soap bars that have extra fats added, such as olive oil, cocoa butter, lanolin and mineral oil. The amount of fatty material depends on the brand, but while normal soap contains 2 per cent fat, superfatted bars contain between 5 and 15 per cent. This improves the soap's ability to moisturise and it is less irritating, so it's a better option for sensitive skin.

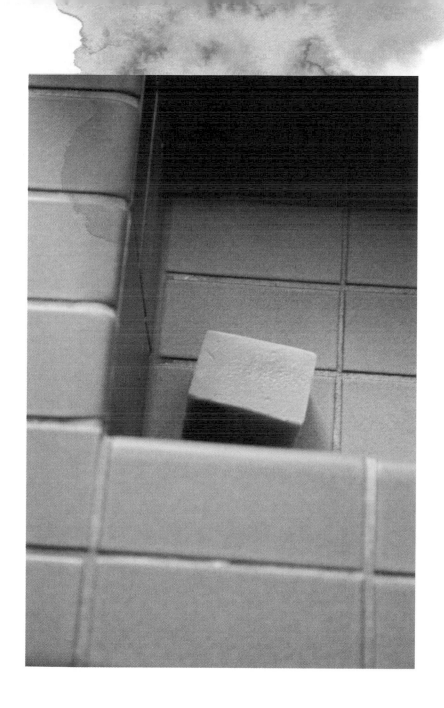

237   Bathe

TRANSPARENT SOAP

This is a special type of superfatted soap. As well as additional fat content, it contains ingredients like glycerin, sugar and alcohol. The glycerin makes the bar soft and clear. These soaps are good for people with sensitive but oily skin, but they tend to lather less well than other types of soap. Some people find these soaps more drying because alcohol may draw water from the skin.

CASTILE SOAP

Originating in the Castile region of Spain, this all-natural, vegetable-based soap's main ingredients are olive and laurel oil. Other ingredients can include coconut, hemp, avocado and walnut. This toxin-free and alkaline soap is environmentally-friendly, safe for children and those with allergies, and incredibly versatile.

SYNDET SOAP

Syndet soap is made from fats, oils and petroleum products that bind together using different methods to ordinary soaps, with the aim of making them milder. The pH of these bars is around 5.5, which is similar to the natural pH of our skin, so they are more skin-friendly than traditional soaps.

AFRICAN BLACK SOAP

Native to West Africa, there are several formulations of African black soap, but the core ingredients are palm tree leaves, dried plantain leaves and cocoa pods, alongside various fats like palm oil, coconut oil and shea butter. This soap is rich in antioxidants and a natural skin cleanser. Gently exfoliating, it is ideal for all skin types.

'There are now soaps for every beauty need, from body-buffing through to skin-soothing, and most are very affordable and beautifully packaged'

Excerpt from 'The Prelude' by William Wordsworth

'The Prelude' is an 8,000-word autobiographical masterpiece that is considered one of William Wordsworth's (1770–1850) greatest achievements. In Book 1: Childhood and Schooltime, the poet recollects some of his earliest memories, including his love for the sounds of the landscape and nature. Derwentwater, which he described as 'The fairest of all rivers' ran across the bottom of the garden where he grew up in Cockermouth, in the Lake District, and he recounts some of his childhood activities, which included playing outside and naked river bathing.

Was it for this
That one, the fairest of all rivers, loved
To blend his murmurs with my nurse's song,
And, from his alder shades and rocky falls,
And from his fords and shallows, sent a voice
That flowed along my dreams? For this, didst thou,
O Derwent! winding among grassy holms
Where I was looking on, a babe in arms,

Make ceaseless music that composed my thoughts
To more than infant softness, giving me
Amid the fretful dwellings of mankind
A foretaste, a dim earnest, of the calm
That Nature breathes among the hills and groves.
When he had left the mountains and received
On his smooth breast the shadow of those towers
That yet survive, a shattered monument
Of feudal sway, the bright blue river passed
Along the margin of our terrace walk;
A tempting playmate whom we dearly loved.
Oh, many a time have I, a five years' child,
In a small mill-race severed from his stream,
Made one long bathing of a summer's day;
Basked in the sun, and plunged and basked again
Alternate, all a summer's day, or scoured
The sandy fields, leaping through flowery groves
Of yellow ragwort; or, when rock and hill,
The woods, and distant Skiddaw's lofty height,
Were bronzed with deepest radiance, stood alone
Beneath the sky, as if I had been born
On Indian plains, and from my mother's hut
Had run abroad in wantonness, to sport
A naked savage, in the thunder shower.

CALM

Final Thoughts

According to my mother, I was an unusual child. Unlike most children, including my two siblings, I LOVED baths. I did not need to be chased around the house buck naked and almost dragged into the bathtub. There was no need for me to be bribed by bubbles or distracted by dozens of rubber ducks and Fisher Price toys (though Three Men in A Tub was by far my favourite) to keep me from jumping straight back out the minute her back was turned to warm the towel on the radiator. Unlike the others, I did not need to be cajoled into the bath and every single night go through the same drama and battle only to immediately realise once immersed in the bubbly warmth, just how wonderful it was in there.

Not me. I couldn't wait to tumble into the tub and mould my hair into pointy alien-y peaks with shampoo, fashion the wet facecloth into a boob tube and make foamy facial hair (who didn't sport a bubble beard?). And finally, when the others hopped out taking their wet limbs and raucous behaviour with them and I had the tub to myself, I couldn't wait to lay outstretched under the water with only the tip of my nose poking out to breathe, my hair fanning out mermaid-like beside me, listening to the beat of my heart amplified by the confined and watery acoustics, my entirety suspended in what felt like an expansive ocean of timelessness. I was in my element.

Perhaps this is why my work has involved a lot of wallowing around the world, though not all without its challenges. I have braved the Baltic after an extended sauna session near Copenhagen, been whipped with birch branches in Russia, lolled until I was prune-like in the Blue Lagoon, Iceland, wild-swum wherever I could, from the choppy Mediterranean in winter in a wetsuit to naked in still, natural Austrian lakes. I have steamed and sauna'd, of the manmade and natural kind. So to this day I'm aghast at people who don't bathe regularly. For me it's the ultimate unquestionable place to get away from it all, requiring the least effort for the most incredible benefits. You just lie there, doing nothing, while underneath the surface body and mind are cleansing, purifying, renewing. It's the ultimate no-questions-asked skive. I could bathe morning, noon and night, and there's no rhyme nor reason nor timing to my bathing habits. I take a bath whenever I fancy it – in preparation for going out, when I come in from a long day, to wake me up, to calm me down. A hot oily bath can make me feel secure when I am anxious, while a salty bath purfies me when I have overindulged (alternated with freezing-cold shower blasts–hopping in and out from the shower to the tub is my ultimate hangover cure!).

A tepid 'sheep dip', as I call it, is a wonderful, transformative beautifier too; a one-pot pit stop where you scrub away dry dead and dull skin, shave legs or any other parts, softening and smoothing skin from top to toe with all manner of oils and spoils, boosting body confidence in five minutes flat. You step out a new person, a layer shed in every sense.

I have cried in the bath, I have laughed in the bath, I have shared a bath and pondered my life and the Universe in the bath. I have drunk Champagne up to my neck in bubbles and I have enjoyed many a morning coffee in the bath reading the paper. One of the most underrated pleasures of a weekend morning is this: A leisurely supping of hot coffee in a warm bath of a sunny Sunday morning. Exquisite, risqué almost… The cheek of it!

So, buy that bath bridge, that mind-altering bath oil, that plush bath mat, that candle (Three Men in A Tub, if you have to) and go ahead and pour yourself some pink champagne, a cold beer, a herbal tea, freshly ground mug of coffee (or heck, just take the whole cafetière with you!). Then grab a book, a magazine or simply the time to do absolutely nothing, close the door and tell that inner child that once you're in, it's really quite wonderful. I promise you, you'll wonder why on earth you don't do it more often…

CONCLUSION

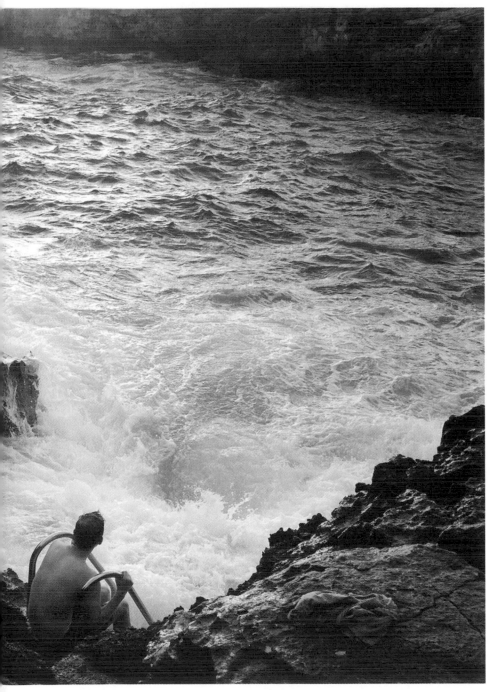

Index

[ITALIC PAGE NUMBERS INDICATE RELEVANT PICTURES]

A

African black soap 238
  (*see also* soaps)
'The Aphrodisiac – for
  romance' 72–3, *73*
  (*see also* recipes)
Archimedes 30
aromatherapy 216–23,
  217, 219, 223
  and bath rules 222
  how it works 218
  popularity of 221
  and South Korean
  research 220, 221
artwork for bathroom 154

B

Bacalar, Mexico 46
balneotherapy 112
banyas 42, 157–8
  as saunas with a
  difference 157 (*see
  also* saunas)
  three rooms in 157–8
  two types of 157
baptism, *see* religious uses
bathhouses 24–5
  oldest 40
bathing accessories, top
  ten 164–5, *165*
bathing and aromatherapy
  216–23, *217, 219, 223*
  and bath rules 222
  how it works 218
  popularity of 221

and South Korean
  research 220, 221
bathroom *155*
  lighting in 154
  paint for 154
  sprucing up 153–5
  technology has no place
  in 191
bathtime:
  before bedtime 215
  brainwaves for 30, 96,
  140, 166, 188, 234
  breathing exercises 90,
  192–3
  and creativity and
  problem solving
  180–3, *181*
  and digital detoxing 191
  and eating and
  drinking, guide to
  172–3, *173*
  and exercises to fuel
  creative thinking 185
  and gong baths
  230–1, *230*
  and music choice 168–9
  reading during
  170–1, *171*
  rituals at, *see* ritual
  short-changed 159
  and simple soaps 236–9,
  237
  and wrinkles 142–3, *142*
  yoga during 126–7
bathtubs 28–9, *29*
bedtime, bath before 215
beer baths 136 (*see also*
  weird baths from
  around the world)

Beethoven, Ludwig van
  166, 169
The Bell Jar (Plath) 146
Biden, Joe 187
Blue Lagoon, Iceland 94
bonding and kinship 16
books, keeping dry at
  bathtime *171*
brainwaves at bathtime:
  from Archimedes 30
  from Beethoven,
  Ludwig van 166
  from Branson, Richard
  96
  from Christie, Agatha
  166
  from Churchill, Winston
  96
  from Ford, Tom 234
  from Franklin, Benjamin
  30
  from Huffington,
  Arianna 188
  from Hugo, Victor 234
  from Mercury, Freddie
  188
  from Winfrey, Oprah
  140
  from Woolfe, Virginia
  140
Branson, Richard 96
'Bring the beach to your
  bath' 60–1 (*see also*
  recipes)
British bathing 44–5, *44*
Buddhism 37, 42 (*see also*
  religious uses)
  and bathhouses 25

C

calmness 206–41, *207*
    and aromatherapy
        216–23, *217, 219, 223*
        (*see also main entry*)
    and bathtime
        brainwaves 234
    DIY recipes for 208–13,
        209, 210, 212–13 (*see
        also* recipes)
    and floatation, joys of
        228–9, *228*
    and gong baths 230–1,
        230
    and natural ingredients,
        twenty 224–7, *225, 227*
    and simple soap 236–9,
        237
'Canon in D Major' 169
Castile soap 238 (*see also*
    soaps)
China, ancient, and
    aromatherapy 216 (*see
    also* aromatherapy)
chocolate baths 136–7, *137,
    139* (*see also* weird
    baths from around the
    world)
Chopin, Frédéric 169
Christianity 37 (*see also*
    religious uses)
Christie, Agatha 166
Church disapproval 25
Churchill, Winston 13, 96
'Clair de Lune' 169
clarity 178–201, *179, 190*
    and bathtime
        brainwaves 188
    and bathtime breathing
        exercise 192–3
    and creativity and
        problem solving
        180–3, *181*
    and networking in the
        nude, Finish art of
        186–7, *187*

'Cleansing and calming
    salts and clay combo'
    62–3, *62* (*see also* recipes)
Cleopatra, Queen 13
'Coconut Oil' 211 (*see also*
    recipes)
Coldplay 169
Coleridge, Samuel Taylor
    198, 200–1
communal bathing 40–3,
    41, 43
'Crazy Little Thing Called
    Love' 13, 188
creative storage 153
Crete, ancient 28

D

'Dancing On My Own' 169
de-cluttering bathroom 153
de la Bonnardiere,
    Jacques 124
Dead Sea 93
Debussy, Claude 169
digital detoxing 191
Diplomatic Sauna
    Society 187
Dunton Hot Springs,
    Colorado 94

E

eating and drinking in the
    bath 172–3, *173*
Edward III 25, 45
Egypt, ancient 24
    and aromatherapy 216
        (*see also*
        aromatherapy)
    'The Energiser' 67 (*see
        also* recipes)
    'Eureka!' moment 30
exercise:
    in bath, for creative
        thinking 185
    hot bath compared
        with 122

F

Fairy Pools, Isle of Skye 47
Feetham, William 26
Finland, and saunas 186–7,
    187
Fisher Price toys 242
floatation, joys of 228–9,
    228
Ford, Tom 234
forest bathing (Shinrin-
    Yoku) 194–7, *197*
Franklin, Benjamin 30

G

Gattefosse, Rene-Maurice
    216
ghassoul ritual 117
Gibran, Khalil 204
'Ginger and Fresh Lemon
    Juice' 213 (*see also*
    recipes)
gong baths 230–1, *230*
Goulding Ellie 169
Greece, ancient 24
    and aromatherapy 216
        (*see also* aromatherapy)
green tea, coffee, sake, red
    wine and ramen noodle
    baths 138 (*see also*
    weird baths from
    around the world)

H

hammam (Turkish bath)
    112–19
    and glow at home 119
Hampton Court Palace 45
Handel, G.F. 169
hardware, updating 154
Henry VIII 45
Hepburn, Audrey 50
Hinduism 37 (*see also*
    religious uses)
Hippocrates 216

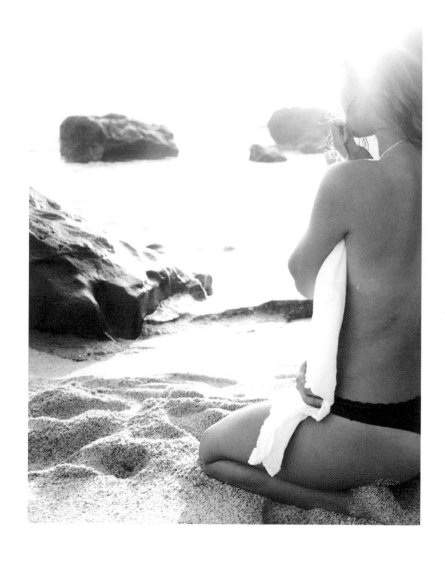

248   Bathe

history of bathing 24–6
hot bath:
    and blood-sugar levels
       112
    and Churchill 13, 96
    and circulation 112
    compared with exercise
       122
    as cure for depression
       108
    and Turkish bath
       (hammam) 42
Hotel Hershey,
    Pennsylvania 136
'How Long Will I Love You'
    169
Huffington, Arianna 188
Hugo, Victor 234

I

I Capture the Castle (Smith)
    108
India, ancient, and
    aromatherapy 216 (*see
    also* aromatherapy)
Islam 38 (*see also* religious
    uses)
Isle of Skye 47

J

Japanese bathing 25, 42
    how to achieve 86–7, *87*
Japanese onsen 42, 74–81,
    75, 76–7, 79, 85 (*see also*
    purification)
    explained 74–5
    not just humans who
      love 85
    sentos versus 80–1
jimjilbang ('heated rooms')
    160–3, *163*
    how-to concerning 162
Jones, Norah 169
Judaism 38 (*see also*
    religious uses)

K

Kawabata, Yasunari 88–9
keeping books dry at
    bathtime *171*
Kekkonen, Urho 186
Kenwood Ladies' Pond 46
Khrushchev, Nikita 186
Knossos 28

L

'Largo' (from 'Xerxes') 169
'Last Request' 169
'Lay Me Down' 169
Layton, Elizabeth 96
Legend, John 169
Leonardo da Vinci 16
'Liebestraum No. 3 in A Flat
    Major' 169
lighting in bathroom 154
Liszt, Franz 169
'The Long Day is Over' 169
Loughborough University
    112, 122
'Love Is a Losing Game' 169

M

'Magic' 169
'magic' time, choosing 151
Mendelssohn, Felix 169
Mercury, Freddie 13, 188
Middle Ages 45
milk for bathing 13
'Moonlight Sonata' 169
Moroccan black soap 236
    (*see also* soaps)
muds, oils and salts 54–6,
    55, 57 (*see also*
    purification)
Muir, John 194
music with bathing 152

N

naked bathing 32–5, *33*
natural ingredients, twenty
    224–7, *225, 227*
networking in the nude,
    Finish art of 186–7, *187*
Nicholls, Wallace J. 176, 180
'On Revisiting the Sea-
    Shore, After Long
    Absence' (Coleridge)
    200–1
Nutini, Paolo 169

O

'Oatmeal and honey' 211
    (*see also* recipes)
oils, muds and salts 54–6,
    55, 57 (*see also*
    purification)
onsen 42, 74–81, *75, 76–7,
    79, 85* (*see also*
    purification)
    explained 74–5
    not just humans who
      love 85
    sentos versus 80–1

P

Pachelbel, Johann 169
paint for bathroom 154
Palace of Westminster 45
pampering yourself 152
    'In the pink' 59, *59* (*see
    also* recipes)
pink salt 59, *59* (*see also*
    recipes)
Plath, Sylvia 146
plumbing 26
poetry, romantic 198–201
    Coleridge 200–1
power baths 54 (*see also*
    purification)
'The Prelude'
    (Wordsworth) 240–1

purification 52–105, *53*
  and bathtime
    brainwaves 96
  and bathtime breathing
    exercise 90
  and detoxing and
    restorative recipes,
    see recipes
  and etiquette 78–9, *79*,
    102
  and Japanese onsen
    74–81, *75, 76–7, 85*
    (*see also* onsen)
  and loneliness 104–5,
    105
  and natural spas 93–5,
    95
  and power baths 54
  and salts, muds and oils
    54–6, *55, 57*
  and saunas 99–103, *101,
    103* (*see also* saunas)
  and skinship 82–3, *82*
  and *Snow Country*
    excerpt 88–9
'Purifying fresh herbs and
  baking soda soak' 64–5,
  65 (*see also* recipes)

Q

quotations from:
  Branson, Richard 96
  Christie, Agatha 166
  Coleridge, Samuel
    Taylor 200–1
  Ford, Tom 234
  Gibran, Khalil 204
  Hepburn, Audrey 50
  Hippocrates 216
  Huffington, Arianna 188
  Leonardo da Vinci 16
  from Muir, John 194
  Plath, Sylvia 146
  Smith, Dodie 108
  Winfrey, Oprah 140
  Woolf, Virginia 140

R

'"Raindrop" Preludes' 169
recipes 58–73
  'The Aphrodisiac – for
    romance' 72–3, *73*
  'Bring the beach to your
    bath' 60–1
  for calmness 208–13,
    209, 210, 212–13 (*see
    also* calmness)
  'Cleansing and calming
    salts and clay combo'
    62–3, *62*
  'Coconut Oil' 211
  detoxing 58–65, *59, 62,
    65*
  'The Energiser' 67
  'Ginger and Fresh
    Lemon Juice' 213
  'Oatmeal and honey'
    211
  'In the pink' *59, 59*
  'Purifying fresh herbs
    and baking soda soak'
    64–5, *65*
  restorative 66–73, *69,
    70, 73*
  'The Reviver – for
    aching muscles' 68
  'The Sleep Inducer – for
    deep and restful shut-
    eye' 70–1, *70*
  'The Upper – for low
    mood' 68–9, *69*
Red Bull Cliff Diving 46
refreshing towels 153
rejuvenation 110–73, *111*
  and bathing through
    seasons 128–35 (*see
    also* seasons)
  and bathtime
    brainwaves 140
  and bathtime yoga
    126–7
  health benefits of
    112–15
  and hot bath compared
    with exercise 122

  and rhassoul ritual 117
  and science of bathing
    112–15
  and thalassotherapy
    124–5, *125*
  and Turkish bath
    (hammam) 116–19, *118*
  and weird baths from
    around the world
    136–9, *137, 139* (*see
    also* main entry)
religious uses 16, 36–9,
  36, 39
'The Reviver – for aching
  muscles' 68 (*see also*
  recipes)
rhassoul ritual 117
ritual 146–73, *149, 150*
  and banyas 157–8
  and bathtime
    brainwaves 166
  and bathtime music
    choice 168–9
  and jimjilbang ('heated
    rooms') 160–3
  personal, creating 151–2
  and seshin (Korean
    body scrub) 163, *163*
  and short-changed
    bathtime 157–8, *159*
  and sprucing bathroom
    153–5, *155*
  and top ten bathing
    accessories 164–5, *165*
romantic poetry 198–
  201
  Coleridge 200–1
Rome, ancient 24, 40
  and aromatherapy 216
    (*see also*
    aromatherapy)
A Room of One's Own
  (Woolf) 140
Russian banyas 42, 157–8
  as saunas with a
    difference 157 (*see
    also* saunas)
  three rooms in 157–8
  two types of 157

INDEX

S

salts, muds and oils 54–6,
55, 57 (see also
purification)
sanitation 26
saunas 99–103, 101 (see
also banyas)
benefits of 100–1
and coals 13
and etiquette 102
Finland loves 186–7, 187
ice bathing after 103,
103
Scott, Calum 169
seasons 128–35
autumn 134–5, 134
and continued growth
132
and hedonistic pleasure
132
and new growth 130
and oil use 128–9, 132,
135
and slowing down 135
spring 130–1, 131
summer 132–3, 133
and taking stock 135
winter 128–9, 129
seshin (Korean body scrub)
163, 163 (see also South
Korean relaxation)
setting mood 152
Sheeran, Ed 169
Shinrin-Yoku (forest
bathing) 194–7, 197
showers:
first, as we know them
26
introduced into homes
26
speed of using 23
Sikhism 38 (see also
religious uses)
simple soaps 236–9, 237

'The Sleep Inducer – for
deep and restful shut-
eye' 70–1, 70 (see also
recipes)
Smith, Dodie 108
Smith, Sam 169
Snow Country (Kawabata),
excerpt from 88–9
snow monkeys 84, 85
soaps 236–9, 237
solo time 22–3, 22
'Songs Without Words' 169
South Korean relaxation
160–3, 163
how-to concerning 162
sprucing up bathroom
153–5
storage, creative 153
Strait of Corryvreckan,
Scotland 46–7
superfatted soap 236 (see
also soaps)
syndet soap 238 (see also
soaps)

T

tattoos 78
technology, no place in
bathroom for 191
temperature, getting it
right 151
Termas Baños de Puritama,
Chile 94
thalassotherapy 124–5, 125
Thermae Bath Spa, Bath 93
'Thinking Out Loud' 169
top ten bathing accessories
164–5, 165
Totumo, Colombia 138
towels, refreshing 153
transparent soap 238 (see
also soaps)
Turkey 42
Turkish bath (hammam)
116–19

U

University of
Wolverhampton 112
updating hardware 154
'The Upper – for low mood'
68–9, 69 (see also
recipes)

V

volcano mud bath 137
(see also weird baths
from around the world)

W

weightless and joys of
floatation 228–9, 228
weird baths from around
the world 136–9, 139
beer baths 136
chocolate baths 136–7,
137
green tea, coffee, sake,
red wine and ramen
noodle baths 138
volcano mud bath 138
wild bathing 46–7, 47
Winehouse, Amy 169
Winfrey, Oprah 140
womb 20–1, 20
Woolf, Virginia 140
Wordsworth, William 240–1
wrinkles 142–3, 142

Y

Yale University 104
The Years (Woolf) 140
yoga at bathtime 126–7
'You & I' 169
Yunessun Spa Resort,
Hakone 138

INDEX

Acknowledgments

The who's who in the book-writing process is very important and deserves your time. It's a public display of thanks, affection and gratitude to the people that together make these brilliant little works of art called books, that you can hold in your hands and that transport you to another mood, another time, another place, perhaps even, help you improve yourself a little.

I'm thrilled you are reading this bit as, by doing so, you are acknowledging everyone's input, so my first thanks goes to you.

The rest of my heartfelt thanks go to the following talented and actually very lovely people who have all played their part brilliantly in creating *Bathe* with me.

I hope you can feel the magic of the synergy and energy that has been put into this book radiating through your fingertips as your turn each page, our collective purpose being: to inspire you, help you feel a little calmer, happier in a complex, busy but beautiful world.

Thank you to the conscientious Oliver Holden-Rea, Senior Editor at Blink Publishing; the encouraging Natalie Jerome, Acquisitions Director and Publisher at Bonnier Books UK; the fantastic, fastidious writer Georgina Rodgers; the artistic, patient Lucy Sykes-Thompson, the designer; and the entire terrific team at Furniss Lawton for their professionalism, support and encouragement, in particular the intuitive Rowan Lawton. You are all my new best bathing buddies, THANK YOU one and all.

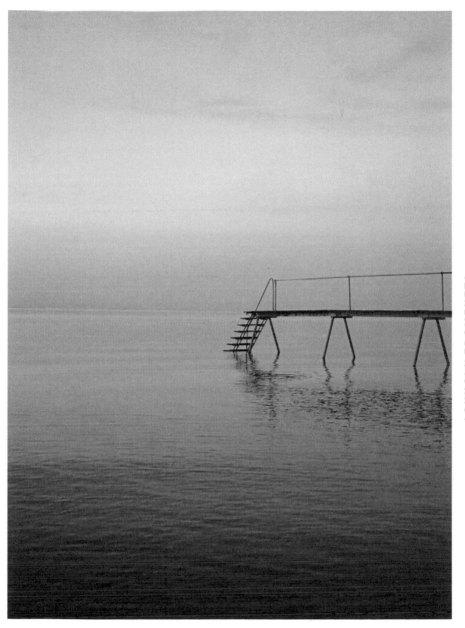

ACKNOWLEDGMENETS

253   Bathe

Photo Credits

p2 Sarah Maingot; p8 Imagery for Sans [ceuticals] Photography: Nastassia Brukin; p11 Imagery for Sans [ceuticals] Photography: Nastassia Brukin; p12 Sarah Maingot, Unsplash/Andrzej Kryszpiniuk; p17 Imagery for Sans [ceuticals] Photography: Nastassia Brukin; p18-19 Sarah Maingot; p20 ©Trinette Reed /Stocksy United, Unsplash/Andrzej Kryszpiniuk; p22 Michael Sinclair/Taverne Agency; p24-5 Unsplash/Tyler Yarbrough; p29 Sarah Maingot; p30 ©Melanie Defazio/Stocksy United, Unsplash/Andrzej Kryszpiniuk, ©Kirstin McKee/Stocksy United; p33 Sarah Maingot; p36 Neale Cousland/Shutterstock.com, Unsplash/Andrzej Kryszpiniuk; p39 Dmitry Kalinovsky/Shutterstock.com; p41 Sarah Maingot; p43 Unsplash/Robb Leahy; p44 Liz Seabrook; p47 Unsplash/Erik Dungan; p53 Sarah Maingot; p55 ©Marti Sans/Stocksy United; p57 Unsplash/Chris Hume; p59 ©Jill Chen/Stocksy United; p.62 Sarah Maingot; p65 Robyn Mackenzie/Shutterstock.com; p69 279photo Studio/Shutterstock.com; p70 Unsplash/Logan Nolin; p73 Unsplash/Masaaki Komori; p75 Lay Koon Lim/EyeEm/Getty Images; p76-77 ©Trinette Reed /Stocksy United; p79 Bhakpong/Shutterstock.com; p82 Sarah Maingot; p84 Imagine Photographer/Shutterstock.com; p87 ©Anwyn Howarth/Stocksy United; p88-89 Unsplash/Michael Xu; p91 Unsplash/Will Swann; p92 Jason Kolenda/Shutterstock.com; p95 Unsplash/Tom Grimbert; p96 © Lauren Naefe/Stocksy United, ©Anwyn Howarth/Stocksy United, Unsplash/Andrezej Kryszpiniuk; p98 Sarah Maingot; p101 Johner Images Royalty-Free/Johner Images/Getty Images; p103 Mika Heittola/Shutterstock.com; p105 Sarah Maingot; p111 Unsplash/Ze Zorzan; p114 ©Trinette Reed/Stocksy United; p118 ©Nadine Greef/Stocksy United; p120-121 Photographer: Alicia Taylor / Stylist: Tigmi Trading; p125 Unsplash/Thomas Peham; p129 Unsplash/Staphanie Studer; p131 Conde Nast; p131 Unsplash/Peter Bucks; p133 Photographer: Alicia Taylor / Stylist: Vanessa Cribb & Caro Toledo / Architect: Angus Munro; p134 Unsplash/Daniel Tseng; p137 Unsplash/Brenda Godinez; p138-139 Unsplash/Tom Crew; p140 © Bonninstudio/Stocksy; Unsplash/Andrezej Kryszpiniuk; © Igor Madjinca/Stocksy United; p142 Sarah Maingot, Unsplash/Andrzej Kryszpiniuk; p149 Unsplash/Hans Vivek; p150 ©Anwyn Howarth/Stocksy United; p155 Sarah Maingot; p156 Deposit Photos; p159 Liz Seabrook for Made.com; p163 Studio Grand Ouest/Shutterstock.com; p165 ©Anwyn Howarth/Stocksy United; p166 Unsplash/Isaac Ibbott, Unsplash/Andrezej Kryszpiniuk, © Giada Canu/Stocksy United; p168-169 Unsplash/Autumn Studio; p171 Photographer: Alicia Taylor / Stylist: Kerrie-Ann Jones; p173 ©Skye Torossian/Stocksy United; p179 Imagery for Sans [ceuticals] Photography: Nastassia Brukin; p181 Unsplash/Lefty Kasdaglis; p184 Sarah Maingot; p187 Westend61/Westend61/Getty Images; P188 Unsplash/Juan di Nella, Unsplash/Andrezej Kryszpiniuk, ©Alita Ong/Stocksy United; p190 Unsplash/Jaz King; p194-195 Unsplash/Aaron Burden; p197 Unsplash/Logan Fisher; p199 Unsplash/Montylov; p200-201 Unsplash/Tom Barrett; p207 Imagery for Sans [ceuticals] Photography: Nastassia Brukin; p209 Michael Sinclair/Taverne Agency; p210 Unsplash/Lindsay Moe; p212-213 Unsplash/Lauren Mancke; p214 ©Daniel Kim Photography/Stocksy United; p217 Unsplash/Norwood Themes; p219 ©Bonninstudio/Stocksy United; p223 Imagery for Sans [ceuticals] Photography: Nastassia Brukin; p225 ©Nataša Mandi/Stocksy United; p227 ©Nadine Greeff/Stocksy United; p228 Liz Seabrook; Unsplash/Andrzej Kryszpiniuk; p230 Unsplash/Manja Benic; p233 plainpicture/Westend61/Oriol Castelló Arroyo; p234 Unsplash/Jack Anstey, Unsplash/Andrezej Kryszpiniuk, Unsplash/Nordwood Themes; p237 Imagery for Sans [ceuticals] Photography: Nastassia Brukin; p240-241 Mike Charles/Shutterstock.com; p244-245 Unsplash/Luke Chesser; p250 Unsplash/Yoann Boyer; p253 Unsplash/Dorini Damsa; p255 Unsplash/Seth Doyle

WATERCOLOUR IMAGES

Elina Li/Shutterstock.com on pages 5, 12, 15, 21, 27, 29, 35, 41, 55, 57, 58, 61, 66, 70, 81, 91, 113, 114, 123, 134, 142, 158, 161, 183, 190, 193, 208, 214, 220, 228, 237, 239; Katerina Izotova Art Lab/Shutterstock.com on pages 17, 39, 137; Anastasiya Samolovova/Shutterstock.com on pages 17, 39, 64, 137, 158; Katya Zlobina/Shutterstock.com on pages 30, 96, 140, 166, 189, 234 Hedzun Vasyl/Shutterstock.com on pages 50, 108, 146, 176, 204; Supa Chan/Shutterstock.com on pages 86, 90, 102, 119, 126, 127, 153, 154, 162, 164, 170, 185, 193, 196, 222

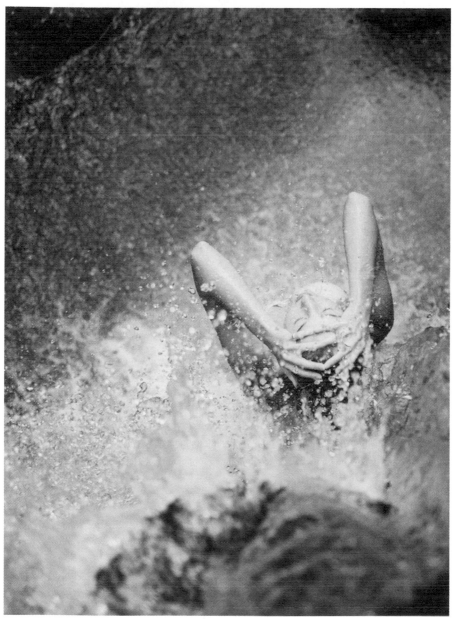

255 Bathe

Published by Lagom
An imprint of Bonnier Books UK
3.08, The Plaza,
535 Kings Road,
Chelsea Harbour,
London, SW10 0SZ

www.bonnierbooks.co.uk

Hardback – 978-1-788700-41-2
eBook – 978-1-788700-42-9

A CIP catalogue of this book is available from the British Library.

Designed by Studio Polka
Illustrations by The Colour Study / www.thecolourstudy.com
Printed and bound by Stige, Italy
1 3 5 7 9 10 8 6 4 2
Copyright © 2018, Suzanne Duckett & Georgina Rodgers

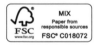